RUNNER'S HIGH

RUNNER'S HIGH

How to squeeze the joy
from every step

JENNI FALCONER

First published in Great Britain in 2024 by Orion Spring,
an imprint of The Orion Publishing Group Ltd
Carmelite House, 50 Victoria Embankment
London EC4Y 0DZ

An Hachette UK Company

1 3 5 7 9 10 8 6 4 2

ISBN (Trade Paperback) 978 1 3987 2089 3
ISBN (eBook) 978 1 3987 2090 9
ISBN (Audio) 978 1 3987 2091 6

Typeset by Goldust Design
Printed in Great Britain by Clays Ltd, Elcograf S.p.A.

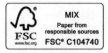

MIX
Paper from
responsible sources
FSC® C104740
www.fsc.org

www.orionbooks.co.uk

This book is for all runners and all the future ones, including my daughter, Ella, who read parts of this book while it was being written and consequently tried out for the cross-country club at school.

CONTENTS

PROLOGUE

I have loved running since my first proper attempt. I was aged nineteen, in Glasgow, dressed in my incredibly stylish 1995 athleisurewear – men's oversized tracksuit bottoms from M&S, some Nike fashion trainers I'd bought on holiday, a long-sleeved Topshop T-shirt and a CD Walkman stuffed in my push-up bra. I had no idea what I was doing, I had little confidence that I was running how 'runners run' and I certainly couldn't maintain even a slow jog for twenty minutes without stopping.

But I was doing it.

I had a burning sensation in my lungs and the back of my throat. It felt like my face was on fire, my hair was glued to my forehead with sweat, my ears were aching from the cold, my legs had acquired a corned beef-style quality and I could feel my heartbeat in every part of my body. I was struggling to catch my breath and anyone passing might have thought I was in pain, yet inside I was beaming because – in actual fact – I truly felt amazing.

That was my first 'runner's high'. On day one!

I had never experienced anything like it. I had pushed myself to complete a run. And, by the way, when I say 'pushed', I mean it, because it wasn't easy. But as I staggered back to my flat, the deep sigh of relief wasn't because it was over: it was total recognition that this running malarky was absolutely, without doubt, my 'thing'.

Since then, running has been more than just a way of staying physically and mentally fit, it's a way of life. It's become part of my lifestyle, a fixture in my schedule, something that I make time for even when there's other stuff I should be doing. Running is one of my priorities because I know the positive impact it has on me, my outlook and my general attitude.

I've created a whole podcast, *RunPod*, that's completely dedicated to just how brilliant and transformative running is. A space filled with the stories of other people who know exactly what I mean when I talk about that 'runner's high'. The absolute joy of running is something that often people do not realise they will experience. I have met a ton of men and women who started running later in life and now wish they'd tried it sooner, but never thought it was for them – how wrong they were!

While I will touch on some of the science behind running and why it makes you feel so good, this book isn't intended to be a scientific guide. It's designed to be a practical handbook, based on my own experience, for anyone at all who wants to start running. An ode to my own running journey, it aims to motivate, inspire and encourage all runners, from newbies and joggers to sprinters, marathoners and endurance runners.

Now, you can read this book from cover to cover and in order if you like. But depending on where you are in your running journey, you may want to dip in and out of the parts that are of most interest to you right now. Chapters 1 and 2 are the ideal starting point for those of you who are completely new to running (or returners who may want a refresher or some ideas to get kick-started). Chapter 5 looks at ramping up your running if you've already started and maybe have your sights set on your first distance target or 5 or 10K race. For more experienced runners, Chapters 6, 7 and 9 look at dealing with the importance of slow runs, navigating runner's lows and of course pushing past your limits. The rest are universal – looking at the science behind the runner's high, the joy of exploring new places while running and what makes our fantastic running community so powerful.

From my own experience, I'll share the highs and lows, the joys and pains, the mishaps and reality checks. I'll bust common myths, share advice and ultimately guide you to getting out there and getting your own runner's high!

The truth is that everyone and anyone can experience

that amazing feelgood effect that comes with running.

You don't have to be a pro athlete.

You don't need expensive kit and gym memberships.

You don't need years of experience.

You don't need to be 'sporty'.

You simply need to do one thing …

Run.

1

TYING YOUR LACES FOR THE FIRST TIME

WHY RUN?

For me, I run because it's my freedom, it's my meditation, it's a chance to reset, feel refreshed, de-stress and get rid of excess energy. If I'm having a great day, it just adds to my buzz and gives me a boost. If I'm feeling low, or irritable, or anxious, I know that even a short run will change my entire outlook, put everything in perspective and help me see clearly again. Of course, these are all my reasons for running *now*. When I first started, I had absolutely no idea these benefits existed. My reason for running then was to lose a bit of weight but most of all to feel healthier.

I saw the benefits really quickly.

Exercising changed my lifestyle completely. I was excited

to get out for a run in the morning, so instead of staying up watching TV until late, I'd go to bed earlier. I wasn't dieting, in fact I was probably eating the same – maybe even more, but it was to fuel my run rather than satisfy my cravings. I was glowing and feeling super healthy but I wasn't restricting or depriving myself, I was just doing something that I was absolutely loving.

Of course, it isn't always plain sailing. In fact, running can bring up some pretty complex feelings. Some days it will feel like a slog and you'll curse every step until it's over. Other days you just won't even want to be bothered and you'll have to force yourself to get out there. Even when you've started, you'll have days when runs don't go to plan. Your laces might be too tight or too loose, you might feel slower, or you'll suddenly need to pee and it completely distracts you. On days like these – and by the way, I do still have them – it's important to focus on *why* you run. This is such a personal thing and it changes over time, sometimes even from week to week, but there is always a reason for running.

When you have one of those bad days, or feel like you can't be bothered, or you're on what feels like a rubbish run, think about just *one* thing you're getting out of that run and focus on what that means to you. Here's a few that I have focused on over time:

☀ A free commute

* Time outside to get some fresh air (no matter the weather)

* Getting a dose of vitamin D on a sunny day

* Thirty minutes on your own to decompress after work or your studies, or a busy day at home

* Thirty minutes to plan ahead for your day

* Thirty minutes to maintain a fitness regime

* Thirty minutes to feel healthier

* Thirty minutes to help you sleep later

* Bragging rights over your partner/friend, who hasn't been for a run!

It helps to look at the bigger picture too. I asked someone once, 'Why do you love running?' and they simply replied: 'Because I can.' It reminded me what a privilege it is to be able to run when so many people who want to can't. Shouldn't we all have this positive approach? Most importantly, when it gets difficult, remember that this is a journey. We're all at different points on that journey and we're all still learning, because with running you only learn by doing it, over and over.

So, keep persevering. Smile, pull on your trainers and take full advantage because it's a gift. Once you realise how the benefits of running can impact your life for the better, you'll never look back. I promise you, the only runs you'll regret are the ones you don't do.

GETTING STARTED

If you've picked up this book, chances are you've heard something about how great running is and you're curious. Maybe a friend has started running and they've been telling you all about it, or you keep seeing people jogging past your bus or car on your commute. You might have run in the past, but then life happened and you just haven't had the time to start again. Maybe glowing, exhilarated runners keep popping up on your Instagram feed, a celebrity you follow has mentioned it as part of their fitness regime, or colleagues at work are taking part in a charity run.

It looks great. It's free. It seems easy to get into. You *know* it's meant to be good for you.

But you've just not acted on it.

I know the exact feeling because I've been there. When I did my first run, I was living between Glasgow, where I worked, and 200 miles away in Leeds, where I studied Spanish, Italian and Latin at Leeds University. I was loving my first ever TV presenting job, travelling around Scotland doing all kinds of crazy, exciting activities, from wood-chipping and skydiving to rock climbing and racing Reliant Robin cars in a BBC Scotland series called *The Big Country*. But I'd experienced a complete lifestyle change. I was busy and doing activities at work but I wasn't being active. I'd gone from being the girl who did all the sports at school, playing hockey and doing Cindy Crawford workout videos at home to being pretty sedentary, driving from shoot location to home and back again, often snacking as I travelled.

Any free time I had was spent getting to know my colleagues or catching up on sleep. Back at uni, I'd be spending time with my friends and flatmates – often in the student union bar, enjoying a pint of Snakebite and Black (cider, beer and blackcurrant for the uninitiated). There was no time at all for exercise. My diet wasn't great, I wasn't active and I'd even started to feel a bit out of place in the clothes I loved to wear. I just felt uncomfortable but more than that, my lack of activity meant I felt sluggish, devoid of energy for anything and just not like myself at all.

I hated that feeling and really wanted to get myself back.

Searching for something that fitted into my schedule, I tried swimming, which was OK, but after doing lengths up and down the pool as quickly as I could, just to get it done, I'd come out and think, *god, that was boring*. Aerobics classes weren't my thing either. Grape-vining and bouncing up and down on a step just gave me a headache and I'd howl 'Nooooo!' internally at the mention of star jumps.

As I tried these things, the idea of running kept popping up. Now, back in 1995, runners weren't as common a sight on the streets as they are now, but I seemed to notice them all the time. In fact, I'd find myself feeling envious that they were out there doing it. I'd see runners on the

5

TV doing marathons too and be in awe that they were all so fit and athletic, and doing something that was a real challenge. Even the guy I was seeing at the time was a runner, training for all kinds of races. But to me, they were *proper* runners. I admired them, but I didn't think I could be like them.

Everything I saw was telling me that running would do what I wanted it to do. It would keep me active without costing the earth, it would challenge me, it would re-energise me and keep me fit and healthy.

But I *still* couldn't get started.

THE FIRST RUN IS THE HARDEST

The truth is your first run is always the hardest. For me, it was the sheer effort that was stopping me. First of all, I lived in a third-floor flat in Hyndland in Glasgow. It was autumn and already bitterly cold outside. If I wanted to run, I'd have to get dressed, get down three flights of stairs, lock up and go out into the freezing cold. Who could be bothered with that? Then there were all the practical questions. What should I wear? Where do I go? Should I go in the morning or the afternoon? Where the hell do I put my keys?! But more than anything, I procrastinated because I didn't know what would happen when I got out there.

I thought my body would wobble when I ran, that I'd be out of breath and that people would be looking at me. The guy I was seeing lived around the corner too and I really didn't want to bump into him like that, so I just kept putting it off. But running kept coming for me. It was a conversation with my boss that finally convinced me. She'd been running for a few months, so I asked about how she was finding it.

'I'm thinking about going running,' I said tentatively one day. 'I like the idea, but it seems hard.'

'Oh, it's great, you should definitely do it,' she insisted.

Then she proceeded to tell me the most amazing story about how her boyfriend at the time was a marathon runner and always used to brag about it. Secretly, when he left for a run, she'd go out running too and make sure she was back before him.

'He'd come back and think that while he was out, I was simply at home sitting on the sofa – little did he know,' she laughed. 'Then, after a few months, I went out running with him and I beat him. It was the best thing.'

As she talked about running, she was positively beaming. She made it all sound so achievable. After months and months of sitting on the idea, it was suddenly like: *OK, I'm listening.*

What was the worst that could happen?

I really didn't have a clue what I was doing, but I picked a day, got up in the morning, grabbed some Nike trainers that I'd bought on holiday and fashioned the rest of my running kit from what I already had in my wardrobe – my normal push-up bra, baggy men's M&S jogging bottoms with a big drawstring waist, socks, a long-sleeved T-shirt and a woolly hat.

I decided to run a route that I would usually walk to the shops, up to Byres Road and around Glasgow's Botanic Gardens, as well as past where my grandma had lived before she'd passed away, because I loved going by her house. After all, if I could walk it, running would be faster, wouldn't it?

I got down the stairs and locked up. Still at a loss as to where to put my keys, I shoved them into one cup of my bra, then stuffed my CD Walkman into the other cup, pressed 'play', walked down my path and just started running.

I took the side streets to Byres Road and it was early, so there weren't too many people around to witness my attempt. Almost immediately, my throat started burning and I was quickly out of breath, but I set my mind on a goal.

I'll just have to get round the Botanic Gardens, that's all, I told myself.

By the time I got to the Botanic Gardens, a few minutes away, the burning in my throat had intensified and spread to my lungs; sucking the cold air in stung as I fought to catch my breath. I wasn't moving fast at all; I could hear the slow slap of my soles on the pavement over a soundtrack of 'Creep' and 'High and Dry' by Radiohead – in stark contrast to my racing heartbeat, which I could feel pulsing in every single part of my anatomy; my throat, my chest, my hands – even my shins were throbbing.

It was hard, it was slow. I was very aware that – bright red in the face and gasping for air – I probably looked like I was in a lot of pain to passers-by. But the strange thing was, I was enjoying it. *Really* enjoying it.

I was outdoors, gulping in fresh, cold air. I was moving, I was active. I felt *great*!

I know now that this was the endorphins, my feelgood hormones, kicking into action. Despite the discomfort, feeling tired and breathless, that buzz drove me to keep on going.

I'm going to do this, I told myself.

My run became a jog, then a stagger, and I stopped to catch my breath more times than I could count. But, eventually, I did it: I had made it all the way round the Botanic Gardens.

I can't remember how long it took me. All I can remember is the sensation I was left with when I got home. Tired, hot and sweaty, I looked anything but attractive, but I didn't care. I was beaming, inside and out. It was like I'd really achieved something, even though I'd run … well, not very far at all. It was a feeling I'd not experienced after swimming or any other fitness class. A sense of pure, brilliant and inexplicable joy – my first ever 'runner's high'. I couldn't wait to get out there again and I couldn't believe I'd put it off for so long.

If there's one thing that I wish I'd known before that first run, it's this: You answer all of your questions by getting out there and doing it. Take my paranoias, for example.

Will I be out of breath? (I was); will my body wobble? (I didn't notice); will I have to stop? (I did); will people look at me? (No); have I got the right kit? (I didn't, my trainers were fashion shoes and eventually gave me shin splints).

The truth is, you learn how to run by doing it and eliminating all the wrong answers. As you do so, it opens up a world of amazing benefits: physical fitness, mental wellbeing, seeing where you live in a fresh light, exploring brand new places, challenging yourself, making new friends … the list is endless. But I don't want you to wait as long as I did for that world to open up so here, I want to share some tips and advice that I wish I'd known so you can get started sooner.

HAVE I GOT THE RIGHT KIT?

The beauty of running is that it's free, you can do it anywhere and you don't need any specialist equipment – so the answer to that question is probably yes. Further down the line, you might find there are things that will make your running experience better or more enjoyable, like clothes made from certain materials, fitness trackers and all the other latest gadgetry, but these are *not* essentials. There really are just a handful of things that you need and most likely, you already have them at home.

Shoes

The only really essential bit of 'kit' for running is a comfortable, well-fitting, well-cushioned and supportive pair of sports trainers. It might seem daft to spell it out as it's kind of a no-brainer, but you'd be surprised how many people go running in Converse or, as I did, in the kind of fashion trainers that look good with jeans or in the pub on a Saturday night but are truly not right for running.

If you have sports trainers and they're comfy, you're on to a good start, but you need to make sure they fit properly. If they are too small or too big, they could rub, which may in turn cause blisters. In fact ill-fitting trainers can lead to a whole load of issues from shin splints to heel pain and even stress fractures. I have experienced some of these and they are no fun at all. Shin splints in particular are pretty common, and is when the muscles, tendons and bone tissue around your shinbone (tibia) become inflamed, making them very painful indeed – not something you ever want and most certainly not when you're just starting out.

Be careful with old or worn-out trainers, no matter how

much you love them, and regardless of how many adventures you've had together, you need to know when to say goodbye. If they are worn out and have covered a lot of miles – it's time to retire them. You can usually tell just by looking at them. By this stage, the chances are all the support, cushioning and the rest of the trainer tech benefits you invested in when you bought them will have worn off so get yourself a new pair – for your feet and legs' sake!

What's more, the soles of old trainers can lose their grip over time, which means you could slip if it's wet underfoot or you run over some grass – falling won't be the ideal start to your new hobby. If you don't own a pair of proper running shoes, or you just need some new trainers, you don't have to invest in expensive or fancy branded clobber, they just need to be a decent pair of all-round sports shoes. Often going for old models in discontinued colours online, will mean the shoe is a little cheaper too. Ultimately, think of it as an investment – even if running isn't something you do forever, your new shoes can be worn for other sports too.

Clothes

Now, once you get the running bug you might find that you show more of an interest in running kit and before you know it, you'll have more clothes for running than anything else (or is that just me?). But for starting out, there are really no rules on what your 'running kit' should look like and it certainly doesn't need to be from a specific running brand.

For years I wore my hair pulled back, a cap (so people couldn't see me), a long-sleeved T-shirt and baggy joggers. I didn't wear leggings or even consider anything remotely form-fitting until I did my first marathon in 2009, almost fifteen years after I'd started running. Looking back, why did I want to conceal everything so much? There was absolutely no reason to do so, but at the time, that was how I felt comfortable and comfort is so important when you're getting started. Leggings, shorts, joggers, T-shirts, vests, hoodies … they all work, as long as they don't rub in the wrong places. Rubbing leads to chafing, which leads to pain, and you'll want to avoid that as much as possible!

Another exception to the 'no specialist kit' rule is a sports bra. Girls, please don't bounce in your regular T-shirt bra or lacy push-up. See every step as a bounce. If you run 10,000 steps, that's 10,000 bounces – think of the damage to your breast tissue without support, not to mention how painful it can be. Again, sports bras don't have to be super expensive. There are lots of lower-priced high street stores with decent sales, so it's easy to pick one up for a bargain – and it can be worn for all sports, so see it as an investment rather than a splurge.

Consider your socks for running too, so that when your feet sweat, they don't rub or get wet. You want a pair that stays up (when you run, you'll soon learn that many,

many socks slide down). Decent socks are not costly but will make a huge difference to your comfort levels. I find that double-layer running socks are particularly helpful in preventing blisters.

You should also think about where you plan to put the essentials that you need to carry. Keys and other valuables can fall out of big, open pockets. My bra solution was certainly not a long-term one. After a few runs I ended up with cuts all over my breasts from where my keys dug in. I was also lucky we didn't have mobile phones back then because I definitely wouldn't have had any cup space left!

If you are comfortable in leggings, there are lots of great styles nowadays that have zip pockets for keys and your bank card or some change, plus deep, stretchy pockets for your phone that make it much easier to keep your things with you. There are also armbands and waistbands with pockets for popping your essentials in. Whichever you choose, the most important thing is that what you are carrying is secure and not moving around. Imagine the noise when running 10km with keys jingling about in your pocket, or loose change clinking as it bounces around in your jacket. My personal recommendation is to use a tight pocket or a fitted pouch that doesn't bounce, is secure and is comfortable to run with.

Water

On my early runs, I didn't take water with me as I was only going a short distance and I didn't like carrying a water bottle as I had nowhere to put it. As my runs became longer, I used public water fountains or even popped into the McDonald's or a café on my route and asked for a glass of water so my hands weren't full.

There are plenty of other things you can do, though. You could take a route where there's a shop to buy a bottle of water on the way, or there are wrist bottles that have a grip for your hand, so it's easy to hold while running. You could even get a small, light rucksack and pop your water and other bits in there, or squirrel a bottle of water behind a tree or wall somewhere on your route – it's entirely down to preference.

Other essentials

Personally, I always take my phone and headphones with me so I can listen to music or a podcast, check Google Maps or make phone calls while I'm out. It helps take my mind off the running too, which can be handy on any hills! I also take some change or my bank card just in case I need to use a public loo, or hop on a bus or tube if I have to end my run early. Lip balm or lip gloss are always good for avoiding dry, chapped lips and if you have long hair, you might want to take a hair tie or band with you too.

I find it quite pleasing to allocate certain items of my

clothing to 'running'. There are some things that, as soon as I pull them on, I just feel ready to run. If you start to run more frequently, having some gear kept for the sole purpose of running helps to get you right into the running mindset.

The seasons and time of day you choose to run might also mean you need a few other bits to make your run a safe and enjoyable one. In autumn and winter (or spring and sometimes summer in the UK), you may need a jacket for rainy days. There are plenty of lightweight ones out there, just check whether it's actually waterproof or just shower-proof – there is a difference and you will soon know about it in a downpour! Also, in winter I'm never seen running without my gloves – I have Raynaud's syndrome, which means that the blood stops circulating in my fingers and they go white and become extremely painful, so forgetting my gloves isn't an option. I even have long sleeves on my jumpers that I can fold round my hands for extra warmth. Then, of course, there's summer. When the sun is shining, don't forget your sunglasses and SPF – especially a balm containing SPF for your lips, which can burn rather easily when sweat dries them out. Finally, if you're running outside of daylight hours at any time of the year, then some reflective clothing is important, even a head torch might be helpful. Alternatively, I have some reflective armbands which are really handy – just pop them on top of your regular kit. When it is dark, you can even switch them on to flashing mode. You can find more on staying safe while running later, on page 70.

BASIC KIT CHECKLIST

As with everything, there *are* specialist items that can enhance and improve your running experience. There are running specific brands for trainers, clothing and more, which of course come with a heftier price tag. We'll come to this in Chapter 5 when we talk about ramping up your running – because you *will* get there – but for now, here's the kit list that will get you started …

Essential

✻ Well-fitting sports trainers

✻ Sports bra

✻ Sports socks (double-layer)

✻ Top – vest, long- or short-sleeved T-shirt, hoodie

✻ Bottoms – leggings, Capri pants or shorts

✻ Lip balm – for cold weather when lips get dried out easily, and with SPF for when it's sunny

✻ Phone and headphones so you can listen to music or a podcast

* If your phone isn't set up to pay for things, then take a bank card or some change in case of an emergency.

Additional extras

* Cap or running beanie hat for cold days

* Hair tie/band

* Reflective clothing and head torch

* Waterproof or showerproof jacket

* Sunglasses

* Sun cream

* Gloves

* Water bottle

WHAT IF I FIND OUT I'M NOT A RUNNER?

Getting your kit ready for your first run is a bit like getting all your new books, diary, erasers and highlighter pens ready for the start of a new job or new school term: everything perfect and pristine. Runners are the same – we all love to get new kit, it's the fun and exciting part ... But don't let it become a way to procrastinate.

Once you've got your kit sorted, it's time to run. Now, I know this can be a big hurdle. In the back of your mind, you're probably still thinking, 'I'm not a runner', 'It's not my thing', 'I'm too self-conscious' or simply 'I can't run'. Believe it or not, I've felt that way too. In fact, I have a confession to make: I haven't *always* liked running. It wasn't *quite* love at first stride.

Why? Two words: Cross Country.

Few of us will have been spared the horror of this dreaded school sports lesson and I'm no exception. I remember vividly leaving the grounds of my school in the west end of Glasgow at the age of ten with my horrible Aertex shirt tucked into my big gym pants, facing what felt like *miles* of running around the streets of Jordanhill.

It was a mainly residential area next to Anniesland in Glasgow, full of beautiful houses, some fancy delis and gorgeous sandstone tenement buildings, many of which were on big hills with what felt like significant inclines (well, I was ten at the time and they all felt like mountains!).

I *hated* it. There was no feelgood sensation, no 'high', just a burning in my throat, frozen fingers and ears stinging with pain. As soon as the ordeal was over, I'd already be dreading the next time. It couldn't have been further from the experience I had later in life. In fact, I hated cross-country running so much that I even wrote to a TV programme that arranged surprises and asked if they could come and pick my group up just past the school gates, then – after an appropriate amount of time – deliver us where the route ended, so we'd look really fast and wouldn't actually have to do the running.

That's how desperate I was not to have to do it.

Now, I'm sharing this story for a good reason. I know that if this was my first experience of running, I'll bet it was yours too, or something similar at least. These early experiences can shape how we feel about running and exercise generally as adults and they only add to that fear of getting started. It can be difficult to shake off those negative experiences and all the things that we tell ourselves as I've mentioned before, like 'I'm not a runner', 'It's not my thing' or simply 'I can't run'. The first thing you have to do is eliminate those thoughts for these are all misconceptions and – I want you to trust me here – running on your own terms is a million miles apart from what you remember about PE at school. And I promise you, you *can* run. It might not come easily or naturally at first, but the first step is understanding that running is a challenge. It may well be a big step outside of your comfort zone and you might have to push past some long-held beliefs about the sport, but it *is* possible.

PLANNING YOUR FIRST RUN

Overcoming that hurdle of getting out on your first run is all in the planning. First, take some time to think about where you might go. Don't worry about how far you're running, just pick a route that you're comfortable with

– round the block, around your local park, to a friend's house for a cuppa, or even just up and down your street.

Once you know where you're going, plan *when* you're going. Telling yourself that you'll go for a run 'this week' won't work. Believe me, there will always be something that pushes it back again if you haven't set specific times. Instead, look at the week in your diary and plan maybe two or three occasions when you will run. Let's allow thirty minutes for the run – that's like an episode of your favourite sitcom, no time at all. This means you could squeeze it in before work or after, or just at some point in your day when you have half an hour free. I always like running on a Monday as it's great to start the week strong, especially if you get out early – you'll feel proud all day and will certainly have earned bragging rights!

When you've picked your days, mark them in your calendar or diary, set an alarm, do whatever you do for important appointments that you have to keep. Make sure you have everything prepared the day or night before. Get all your kit washed and laid out wherever you get ready so you don't have to spend time rooting around for clean pants or searching for an errant trainer – you can just get dressed and go. And by the way, you don't have to run every day. In fact, allowing yourself a rest day in-between gives the body time to recover and a day for you to mentally get excited about improving on your last run!

Activity: Plan your first run

Write down your first running plan and stick it to the fridge, mirror or somewhere you can see it and get excited about it. Remember:

* Set a specific day and time for your run

* Work out how much time you have for your run

* Plan your route – where will you go, based on the time you have available?

* Put it in your diary or calendar with the time you need to set off

* Lay your kit out ready the day or night before

* Set your alarm, with snoozes if you need them!

Here's an example:

Monday
Get up and run. An easy run would be 7–7.30 a.m. Run to the park and back.

Tuesday
Day off. Organise your kit for Wednesday's run.

Wednesday

Get up and run before work or whatever you have planned for the day (6.30–7.15 a.m.). Run to the hill; do hill repeats (repeat runs) x five (run up, walk down), run home again.

Thursday

Day off. Message friends (if you have running buddies) to confirm Saturday morning's run.

Friday

Day off. In the evening, get your kit out for the parkrun tomorrow. Parkrun is a free, community event where you can walk, jog, run, volunteer or spectate. Check online for details of this 5K run that takes place every Saturday morning (and see also page 198).

Saturday

Early-morning 5K parkrun.

Sunday

Day off, but remember to put your kit out that night for your Monday run!

On the next page, you will find a grid that you can photocopy to fill out your own plan. You could even file copies of your plans to keep a record of your progress.

GETTING IT DONE: YOUR FIRST RUN

You've got your kit, planned your route and you know when you're going to run. All that's left is getting it done.

It's the most important thing, but it's also the most difficult thing.

The thing is you don't *actually* have to run your first run. In fact, this is something that I've recommended for listeners on my podcast, *RunPod*. Even if you just walk your route, on the day you planned to do it, you've still gone out there and done it. It might even help you to feel more confident next time, knowing your route better. You see, you have to set your own level and if, for you, that's a walk around your chosen route, then that's great. That's your first run and your level set. Now you just have to build on it.

If it takes you ten minutes walking it the first time, set yourself a goal for the next time; challenge yourself to do it quicker. Next time, add in a short jog or run. Completed it in nine minutes and forty-five seconds? Congratulations, that's your first personal best (PB) right there!

After my first run, which, by the way, I walked quite a lot of, I challenged myself to do it a bit faster the next time.

Mon	Tue	Wed	Thur	Fri	Sat	Sun
AM						
PM						

All I really wanted was to get to a point where I could run that route, the whole way, without stopping. But that was going to take time.

When I started running, my level was a very stop-start jog around the Botanic Gardens. Every run I did, my aim was to run for a bit more of the route each time. It didn't even have to be much more, as long as it was more. It took me two whole months to be able to run around the Gardens competently and confidently without stopping. Even then, I wasn't fast; I just didn't stop. I didn't notice it becoming easier, but it must have been, because I was able to run more each time.

The high from those little successes was incredible. After each run I was buzzing – I thrived on the red face, the blood rushing to my thighs and giving my skin that corned-beef effect! I adored the sensation of getting into a hot shower when I was still cold from being outside, I loved that first glass of water when you get back to the kitchen. But more than all that, I also loved the fact I felt so, so amazing. I'd smile, start thinking about when and where I would run next time … and I'm still like that today!

A NOTE ON WARMING UP, COOLING DOWN AND STRETCHING

I did yoga classes for years and still do occasional Pilates, but I stopped stretching directly before a run because I was told it was in vain. Warming up before a run is a good move, but contrary to popular belief it does not necessarily involve stretching. There is actually *no* evidence that pre-run stretching is beneficial and in fact there are those who claim it is quite the reverse. It does not prevent injury nor improve performance and there is even evidence that static stretching (where you hold a single position for a period of time) has a negative impact.

Instead, to warm up pre-run, try some gentle jogging or drills such as walking with the hip out, then hip in, side-stepping, skipping with high legs, lunge walks … There are plenty of options. It's about raising the heart rate and getting the blood pumping.

A post-run cool-down is also a good idea. That could be some long hold stretches (hold for at least thirty seconds and don't move too quickly through them), or even an ice bath (see page 117). A cool-down can help regulate your heart rate after a hard run, it can help reduce the build-up of lactic acid, which can cause muscle fatigue and soreness and it helps the body relax too.

BREAKING IT DOWN

A great way to build up progress is to break your run down into 'intervals'. This is simply running for a set amount of time before a brief period or 'interval' of walking or running at a slower pace. Try walking for your first minute, then running the next twenty seconds, then walking the next minute, running for twenty seconds, and so on and so forth. You could do this for the duration of your planned route, or set an amount of time, such as twenty or thirty minutes. The aim is to reduce the walking and up the running a little bit each time, so once you've cracked walking for one minute and running for twenty seconds, change it up. Walk for forty seconds and run for thirty seconds instead, building up gradually so you're running more and more each time. It's these small incremental goals that will keep you progressing *and* buzzing for your next run.

Once you're running most of the way, you could set yourself the challenge of reaching a point (or series of points) along your route where you stop for one minute. As you catch your breath, use the time to reflect on how brilliantly you have done to make it to that point, before starting again. Once you can do that, see if you can do it a little quicker, maybe lose a stop point or two, or even shorten your rest time. Before you know it, you'll be running the whole way and you may even do what I did, adding on distance when I felt I could - an extra street here, an additional right turn there – all the while building your ability and stamina.

Running is a personal journey – if you take small steps and make gradual progression, you'll see huge improvements in everything from your physical fitness to your mental wellbeing. Whatever you do, and however you get started, it's important to always be keen to build on the last time or challenge yourself a little more – that's part of the fun! It will not be easy and you may even question why you're doing it while you're running. However, I guarantee that once you're home, all sweaty and glowing, your runner's high will remind you. The self-satisfaction and pride will kick in and by the time you have your breath back, you'll be thinking about how you can do that little bit better next time. Of course, whenever you're learning to do something new, there will be worries and bumps in the road, which I think it's important to talk about here.

WILL EVERYONE BE LOOKING AT ME?

The really short answer to this is no. It's completely understandable to feel exposed and on show when you're taking yourself out of your comfort zone and pushing yourself. You're filled with self-doubt, you're worried about jiggling and sweating and being slow, and you don't want anyone to see it. But there's really nothing at all to worry about.

There are two groups of people that bother those new to running: people who are already 'runners' and those who aren't. So, everyone, basically. Speaking as an existing member of the running community, I know that I do look at other runners. But if I look, I'm probably just jealous that they're out running, thinking about my next run, or maybe admiring their leggings. You see, the moment you step out for a run, the very second your foot hits the pavement, you're in the gang. If you clock a look from another runner, whether a hobby jogger or elite marathoner, it will be one of acknowledgement. If another runner runs past you, that doesn't mean you're rubbish, they won't be judging you. Remember, they were you once upon a time. Now you're one of us, a member of the running community, and we all have one another's back. And as for everyone else going about their day? Chances are they're staring into space or looking at something else. But if not, who cares? Are they running? No, they're not. You are, though – you're making that effort.

You're already one up on them.

Another thing to remember is when people see you running, they have no idea how long you've been running *for*. If someone sees you wheezing five minutes into a jog round the park, they don't know you've only been running for five minutes – for all they know, this could be your hundredth lap! However, if you are still super conscious about people seeing you running, there are ways around it. For a long time I hid under my cap or woolly hat so people couldn't see me. Sticking to side streets rather than main roads or pathways is also a good way to dodge lots of people too.

Timing your run can also help. Getting up and out early in the morning is always a good option because you're done before the commute and the school run even starts. Similarly, later in the evening when everyone has headed home is much quieter. But funnily enough, not long after I started running, I actually started picking routes with *more* people on them. Roads where people would be milling about and I felt safer, and even past the then-BBC building on Queen Margaret Drive, where some of my bosses were based. You see, I found that I was far less likely to stop if people could see me and being around people gave me the drive to keep moving.

Maybe you can turn your fears and worries into a motivator too?

WHAT IF I CAN'T STICK TO IT?

A great way to get started *and* stick to your plan is involving your friends, family or even colleagues. Now, you can run together if you want, but you don't have to. If you can, then great, you'll have one another for moral support and, of course, safety. But another way to involve others is to agree to a run challenge that you set between yourselves that you can do together – but apart – because goodness knows, getting people together at the same time can be a challenge in itself!

Create a WhatsApp group and share the target for the week, let's say three, thirty-minute runs. Everyone decides their own time and place, but they all have to share their plans and report back into the group once it's completed. Let the group know when each run is done and how it went – you could even send a post-run selfie. Being accountable to others like this can be a perfect way to commit to running, but it's also an opportunity to share the ups and downs, work out how to navigate challenges together and to have a gang to celebrate those little successes with.

RUTH'S STORY

If you need some more inspiration to get started, then Ruth Langsford is it. In December 2021 the TV presenter came on *RunPod* to tell me all about her Couch to 5K journey. She said: 'I found it really hard but it's such a fantastic feeling when you start off and you're just running for one minute and you're thinking, "Oh god, I can't do this." Then all of a sudden, you're doing twenty and you think, "Crikey, four or five weeks ago I struggled to run three minutes, now I'm running twenty non-stop" and there's that feeling of achievement.

'It also made me want to eat healthily, because if I'd been out for a run I wasn't going to come back and eat loads of toast and butter, I was going to have a protein smoothie. It helped everything in my life.'

Ruth told me how using the NHS Couch to 5K app to get started made her realise what was actually possible. 'I think it's an amazing idea – it talks you through, encourages you,' she said. 'The little steps you build up and build up and then you think, "Gosh, my body really can do this".' What she hadn't bargained for was the mind games required to motivate herself to run, but fortunately, some friendly advice helped her through. She explained: 'My friend said to me, "When you know you're going to do your run, put your running kit on straight away when you get up. It shows intent. Even if you don't go then until four o'clock in the afternoon, even if you do 101 other things, it shows intent" and I realised once I was out the door, I was actually all right.

'The feeling of achievement, of self-satisfaction and even smugness when you've done it, whether it's a minute or thirty minutes, you feel so proud of yourself. When they say about endorphins released, I absolutely get that – I did feel fantastic, every single one I completed. I was so proud of myself.'

Activity: Set a running challenge

It can be hard to know exactly what kind of challenge to set for yourself at the start, and there's enough to think about with just getting yourself into the habit of running. So, to make it easier, here's an example to get you started ...

* Challenge One – Move for thirty minutes non-stop – it doesn't matter what distance you do or if you walk, run or jog, it's just about moving for thirty minutes non-stop.

* Challenge Two – Run five minutes, then walk for two minutes. Repeat this three times.

* Challenge Three – Do a 5K, (a parkrun for example, see their website for details) running as much of the distance as you can.

TAKE THE *RUNPOD* 5K CHALLENGE

Ruth took on the Couch to 5k Challenge, surprising herself and achieving what plenty of people believe is impossible – that we *can* actually run. So, if Ruth can, why don't you try working up to your first 5K, using the *RunPod* 5K Challenge on page 257?

Devised by celebrity trainer 'Mr PMA', Faisal Abdalla, with a little help from myself, it will get you running a 5K, all in one go. You can follow the plan from the book or get encouragement and be entertained by running while listening to the podcast episodes.

2

FINDING A ROUTINE THAT WORKS FOR YOU

So, you're over the hurdle of getting started and you've realised that this running lark is actually pretty great. You want to keep going, but now you're facing a new challenge: when do you fit it in? You might have done everything that we covered in the previous chapter – picked your route, decided what days to run and got your kit and flat-laid it out, so you're ready to go – but plans can easily go awry as life happens around you. A closed road on your planned route or a missing shoe just before you head out can all threaten to set you off-track. Or just managing to fit it in between work or studying, looking after a family, other hobbies or keeping up with your social life can leave you feeling like there's just no time to do it.

The truth is that there is *always* a way to squeeze a run

in, but when we're flying around being busy, it can be hard to see exactly when. Also, like getting started, if you try and do it on the fly, I can guarantee it just won't happen – there will always be something more important that crops up. Scheduling in your runs isn't just a box-ticking exercise, it's about honouring a commitment to yourself to do something that makes you feel good, improves your physical and mental health, and helps you to work towards your personal goals.

SETTING PERSONAL GOALS

We all have different reasons for running. They might be working up to a 10K race, losing weight, improving your mental wellbeing, or simply maintaining good health and fitness levels. These are all known as 'outcome goals' – the overarching result that we want to achieve.

Outcome goals are great – they allow you to broadly assess your overall performance and improvements – but they're not very easy to measure. As well as having outcome goals, it's important to have 'process goals'. These are basically activities that will contribute to your overall goal, broken down into manageable steps. What's more, they're 100 per cent controllable by you.

To set a process goal, look at the outcome you want to achieve, work out what steps you need to take to achieve that, then plan each one in. So, let's say the outcome you want is improving your general level of health and fitness and that you want to do that through running. NHS guidance currently recommends 150 minutes of moderate physical activity per week. To achieve your desired outcome, you need to do 150 minutes of running per week.

Now, technically, it's possible to do just that in one go. But is it realistic? If you're newish to running, it's likely to be a bit too much physically, but more than that, if you're busy, it's too big a time commitment for one day. You're also unlikely to meet the 150-minute target if you just try and wing it and do a few minutes here or there, without a plan in place. What you need is a process goal that is specific, measurable, achievable, relevant and time-bound, or 'SMART' for short!

A SMART goal in this situation might look something like this:

'Each week, I will do three thirty-minute runs between Monday to Friday, and one sixty-minute run at the weekend.'

This is relevant to your overarching goal, measurable, time-bound to each week and far more specific than a vague 'I will run 150 minutes each week'. It's also so much more achievable.

Of course, this is just an example based on national guidance on activity levels for a healthy lifestyle. At first, 150 minutes of running per week could feel way out of reach, so your goals might start smaller and build up. You could start by walking for those 150 minutes each week or running for just ten minutes of each of your thirty-minute runs and walking the rest. Where you start and how you break it down is entirely up to you. This goal-setting strategy just provides you with a framework to work with. Once you know what you need to do to achieve your goal, you can set about planning it in far more easily.

CREATING A TRAINING SCHEDULE

The best advice I can give you is to plan your runs in as you would any other important appointment, like a meeting with your boss, a doctor's appointment or dinner with your best friend. Look at your diary and see where you might be able to fit those three thirty-minute runs into your week and where you'll be able to do that longer weekend run. For example, I try to do this with my runs before the start of each new week. I know that I need an hour and a half to do my run and fit in a shower before whatever is next on my list, so I'll look at my diary, find where I have the time and I write each run in as an appointment.

As a presenter on Smooth Radio, I'm on-air from 6 a.m.

until 10 a.m. so my day starts *really* early. On a standard, term-time workday for me, my alarm goes off at 4 a.m. Then again at 4.15 a.m., 4.20 a.m., 4.25 a.m. – before I eventually stop hitting 'snooze' and get up at 4.30 a.m., which gives me time to get showered, dressed and in work ready to start my show. Running home after work is what suits me best, so I'll go into work in my running gear (which I'll have laid out the night before), leaving the house around 5 a.m., allowing me enough time to get to the studio to start my show on Smooth Radio at 6 a.m.

I'll come off-air at 10 a.m., maybe have a meeting or two, possibly record an episode of *RunPod*, then I'll run my commute, getting back home just before lunchtime. After that there's calls to make, maybe recording more podcasts, a game of golf once a week and the school run, followed by dinner and then winding down for the day before I go to bed around 9.30 to 10.30 p.m.

Of course, it's not always that easy. Some days I'll wake up and panic that I've planned wrong. My absolute nightmare is going into work in my running gear, only to find out that I have an important meeting or event that I need to be wearing proper clothes for. This means I'll often second-guess myself, so if you're anything like me, you might want to plan in a few minutes for a pre-run faff! Sometimes, as well, I'll go to work in my running kit, but not quite think my accessories through. Not so long ago I went into work dressed to run home but instead of my backpack, I picked up a fancy over-the-shoulder handbag – I looked fine on the tube in, but quite a sight running home with it clamped under my arm, let me tell you.

There will also be days when my meetings end up taking longer than expected and instead of running straight home, I'll have to run to collect my daughter Ella from school instead. The good thing is, if you're planning ahead, you'll be able to navigate these things rather than have them crop up on the day and throw you off-track.

Once it's in the diary, it's a date. I treat my running session like I would any other appointment in my life – I get there on time and don't let it overrun so I can get to my next commitment as planned. I will also do everything in my power not to change the runs I have booked in. Unless it's absolutely necessary, I will just say that I'm busy at that time and try to find a different time, rather than cancel. If it's something that I do need to do though, I will try and find a way around it. Can I have the appointment at home on a video call? If I do need to be there, in-person and suited and booted, can I bring my running gear in a rucksack and change in the bathroom so I can still run home? Wherever it fits in your day, honouring that commitment to yourself by making non-negotiable space in your schedule is the first step towards finding a routine that works for you.

FINDING CREATIVE SOLUTIONS

If you're still looking at your diary and thinking, *I just don't have the time*, you might need to look closer and get a little more creative. Think of running outside of the 'doing sport' box.

Way before I thought of running as a hobby, I realised that I actually ran *everywhere*. Not put-your-kit-on-and-go-for-a-run running, but almost subconscious running. In school, when one class ended, I'd leap up from my desk and run to the next class. I literally can't remember a time when I didn't get stopped by a teacher shouting, 'Don't run in the corridor!'

Between the ages of sixteen and eighteen, I had a Saturday job in a pub and I'd run just to get there faster. At the end of my shift, I'd run home because I was scared of the dark – all just in my work uniform.

I'm more aware of how useful this is now. Which is good because I cram my diary full and no matter what I'm doing, I always want to do it quicker. I once said in an interview: 'If you want to get something done, ask a busy person' and my family have taken the mickey out of me for this relentlessly since then, but I stand by it. I'm more efficient when I'm busy and running everywhere helps me keep the momentum – the minute I sit down, I don't want to get up again!

Think creatively about when running might actually

support your schedule. If you need to go to the shop to pick up some bits for dinner, why not pop a rucksack on and run to and from your local supermarket? Obviously not one for when you need to do your weekly big shop, or you'll end up needing a cab back, but for a few essentials, this is multitasking at its best!

If you get home and put dinner in the oven, what are you doing during the forty minutes it takes to cook? If the answer is flicking on the TV and channel hopping, or scrolling through social media, could you maybe ask someone to keep an eye on your dinner while you go out for a quick run then? (I promise you that a twenty-minute run will leave you feeling a million times better than a deep-dive into the comments of a random Facebook post.)

If you're a parent, I also highly recommend running with your little one in a running buggy. Advice says that once a baby is old enough to sit up and hold their head up (around six to nine months old) you can run with them, provided your pram is fit for purpose. We had a mountain buggy pram – a three-wheeler pram designed for parents who like running and going off-road. It's like the Jeep of the pram world and it was amazing! Ella absolutely loved looking out as we zoomed everywhere. The pram was so light and the best part – you could carry stuff too – not just things for Ella but water and snacks for me too, you could even stop at the shops and carry extra bits home!

RUNNING TRAINING DRILLS

Thinking about the type of run that you might be able to fit in is another way to get around a packed schedule. If you're relatively new to running, the only type of run you might know is the route you do regularly, but there are other ways:

Hill sprints – Basically, intervals with an incline. Find a hill that's convenient for you to get to. Run up the hill. Jog or walk down the hill. Repeat. You can set the number of repeats you do, or do as many as you can in the time you have available in your diary.

Repeats – Pick a short distance that's manageable in your time frame, say 400 or 800 metres (or just choose two points a reasonable distance apart to run between) and run it multiple times. You could run between trees in a park or up a nearby road, wherever is convenient. Beginners may want to start with two or three repeats and build up from there.

Fartlek – 'Fartlek' means 'speed play' in Swedish and is a technique in which you alternate between sprinting, jogging and walking. You can do longer sessions, but a twenty-minute Fartlek session might look something like this:

Warm up – Five minutes, very slow run
Set – Run hard for one minute, then jog/walk for one minute. Repeat x six
Cool down – Three-minute jog/walk.

TEMPO RUNS

Tempo runs or 'threshold runs' as they are sometimes called, are training at the fastest pace you can sustain for a long period. Basically, it's how to get a steady speed into your running routine and when you start looking at races, these runs will determine your race paces for 10Ks, half marathons and full marathons. They're pretty gruelling, but also really beneficial.

Now the difference between tempo pace and, say, your absolute fastest pace lies in the science. When you run, the body produces lactate – the product of aerobic metabolism in the muscles. At a tempo pace, your body can process the amount of lactate you produce. Beyond that it can't keep up and you can get fatigued.

You can do a tempo run session in twenty to thirty minutes. I'd suggest something like this:

✳ Brisk walk for two minutes to warm up

✳ Run as fast as you can comfortably for twenty minutes

✳ Slow run for two minutes to cool down.

With different types of runs at your disposal, you'll be able to look at your diary and find more ways to squeeze in a cheeky run. Perhaps you can get off your bus a few stops early and use a long street for repeats? Or arrive early for pick-up, park at the bottom of a nearby hill and do as many hill sprints as you can before the school bell goes?

THE CURSE OF PARENTAL GUILT

Now, unless you're a parent, guardian or carer, this bit will not apply to you, so feel free to skip it if you want. That said, most of us have some form of caring responsibility that will leave us feeling guilty for going out for a run.

As a mum, I know it can be really hard to take the time for yourself when you have a family to look after. This applies to people with caring responsibilities as well. With children, often, it's easier when they are very young – they sleep a lot, are happy to go to the other parent or a family member, or you can buddy up with someone with kids of a similar age. As they get older, though, they might get upset when you leave the room, call for you as you're heading out, or even beg to go with you. I think every parent knows what that tug on the heartstrings feels like – it can be *awful*. But it really is just a few minutes and it's good for children to learn a little bit of independence when you go out. And, oh my goodness, how valued do you feel when you come back and they're delighted to see you?

Look at it like this: by leaving the children with another parent, a friend or a family member to go for your run, you are taking twenty or thirty minutes to make yourself a better parent. In taking that time away from your caring responsibilities you are topping up your own cup, so you have something to give to the person or people you look after. You're out in the fresh air, blasting away the stresses of the day, re-energising yourself and putting things in perspective. When you come back, you'll be seeing and thinking clearly, ready to spend quality time with your family without feeling irritated or stressed. It's only a good thing.

You're also setting a great example for little ones. This is so important because data from Sport England's 2022 Active Lives Children and Young People Survey shows that 53 per cent of children are still not meeting the UK Chief Medical Officers' guidelines of taking part in an average of sixty minutes or more of sport and physical activity a day[1]. Of course, there are many reasons why children don't engage in physical activity and they can't be tackled by encouraging exercise alone. But if they see adults around them – particularly parents – making time for exercise, they learn from it and are more likely to be encouraged to be active.

I certainly learnt it from seeing my dad going to football regularly and Mum doing her exercise videos and always encouraging me to try everything from gymnastics to dance. For me, I always wanted my daughter Ella to see me being an active parent and having those routines too. For pretty much every day of her little life, since she was about five years old, she joined me in my evening routine of putting my clothes out for the next day's run, creating a little flat lay of her own with mine. Of course, I'd always come in and change it, but it built those habits and although she's not a runner, she does love swimming and gymnastics! So, if you're ever feeling the guilt about making time for your run, think of these important benefits and remember that you can't pour from an empty cup. If running is what fills your cup, then you should definitely do it – it will benefit you *and* your loved ones.

LIFE HAPPENS, BE KIND TO YOURSELF

No matter how much planning you do, there will be times when things crop up and your training schedule will get disrupted. Illness or injury, the school holidays, a big work or essay deadline or even a dreaded call from nursery, they're all part of life. You might even just be too tired and what you need to do right at that moment is sit and relax. These things happen and that's OK.

When something happens that means I can't do a planned run, it is frustrating, but I have a way of looking at it. Running is something I choose to do for my wellbeing and enjoyment, but it doesn't pay the bills and the world won't end if I miss it (no matter how much my mind argues otherwise!). When you miss a run, if you want to fit it in elsewhere, by all means try. But if you're looking at your diary, trying to find space that isn't there and it doesn't happen, don't worry – you've given it your best shot.

The temptation at this point to get home, cosy up and eat a whole pack of biscuits is real. Of course, you're entitled to do that every now and again, particularly after a really rubbish day. But if the only thing that's happened is that you didn't make one run, don't let it get you down. Dust yourself off, try to leave a few digestives in the packet for another day and see if you can find something else to squeeze in to ease any feelings of annoyance and disappointment.

For example, you could:

* Get off your train/bus a stop or two earlier and walk

* Walk somewhere you'd usually drive/get public transport to

* Commit to getting your daily steps for the day

* Take the stairs in work instead of the lift.

When running becomes part of your life and you build

a routine, disruptions can be hugely frustrating. But in life there are many other things that have to happen too, so you shouldn't be too hard on yourself – you won't suddenly become unfit or forget how to run and there are plenty more days ahead. However sorely I miss it when I don't get the chance to run, I know that very soon the opportunity will come again. When it does, I'll probably struggle at first, but once I get going, I'll be *super* happy. So, let it go, set your sights on your next run and think about how good it will feel when you do it!

KNOW YOURSELF – WHAT KIND OF RUNNER ARE YOU?

As a morning person, I know it's easy for me to say, *but* if you can get out for your run at the start of your day, you'll find it much easier to build a regular routine. Doing it first thing, rather than later in the day when you might be starting to feel tired, or when unexpected tasks could crop up, means you're less likely to put it off or procrastinate. That said, you have to work out what time works best for you.

If you're really not an early bird, or you have too much on already in the mornings, maybe a run at lunchtime will work for you? Lots of people spend a few minutes eating, then spend the rest of the lunch-hour scrolling on the internet or killing time in other ways because often there isn't enough time to do much else. If your work has shower facilities, why not get out there and run for twenty minutes? You could be back at your desk with time left to grab a sandwich! If you have more time at the end of the day and you know that if you sit down on the couch, you won't be getting back up, why not go home via a park and run there, or pop into a local gym and do half an hour on the treadmill before making your way home for the evening?

In some cases, running during the week might actually be impossible, so why not look at what you can do at the weekend? Although plenty of us like to get a few runs in each week, there's no rule that says this is more effective than opting for one big run at the weekend. In fact, a recent major study published in the *JAMA Network Open*, a medical journal published by the American Medical Association, showed that people who fit their weekly recommended amount of exercise into just a couple of days – for example, over the weekend – have a similarly low risk of heart disease and stroke as those who spread it throughout the week[2].

When training for a marathon, I might have to fit some of my longer runs in at the weekend, but as a general rule Sundays are my day off. That's my day to sprawl on the couch, relax and do as little as possible, so I can set myself up for the rest of my busy week. But that's just me, Sundays might be your perfect running day.

Finding out what works for you is a personal journey and you may have to try a few different things until you find your routine. You might also want to consider what *type* of runner you are. By this I mean what's your running style (see below) because it could well have an impact on what works for you.

TERMINATOR OR TIP-TOER: WHAT'S YOUR RUNNING STYLE?

According to my neighbour, who regularly sees me flying past his house, I run like the Terminator – head down, arms swinging, the thump of my steps audible from miles away – and there I was, thinking I glided along gracefully … Since he told me this, though, I've realised he's right and I've noticed plenty of other Terminators charging down streets, around parks and at races. We're everywhere. But we're not the only ones – in fact, there are some common running styles that I have seen pop up everywhere and now I just can't un-see them. So, which one is most like you?

The Plodder
The runner with no reason to run fast, they just want to get where they're going and enjoy the journey along the way. Usually they have a slow, steady stride and might even

stop to smell the flowers or take in a lovely view. They may not run fast or far, but they're running and that's reason to celebrate.

If you're a Plodder, try: A long, relaxing run somewhere there's lots to see. A sprawling park, a stately home with gorgeous grounds, or a vibrant, busy urban area so you can really unwind and enjoy the sights, sounds and smells.

The Shuffler

Similar to The Plodder, The Shuffler isn't fast, but they *can* shuffle a long way. Small, swishy steps are a trademark and they just keep on going. Endurance is their forte!

If you're a Shuffler, try: Signing up for a longer-distance race like a marathon. Use your shuffling skills to achieve something you might not have thought was possible.

The Terminator

This runner pounds the pavement, thumps on the tread-mill and runs with purpose. They're on a mission and you can hear them coming – and they're coming fast! If their head isn't down, they'll be staring straight ahead, completely focused on whatever their goal is.

If you're a Terminator, try: Any run with a goal, a run home, a run to work, a run to the shops, a run for the bus. A run to give your mind space to plan a project. Whenever you run, run with purpose!

The Gazelle

This is the runner that I *thought* I was. They sprint along elegantly, barely breaking a sweat and make running fast look effortless. These runners can carry on for miles and miles, flying up inclines and gliding down hills.

If you're a Gazelle, try: Trail running, you're built for it. Get out in nature, in the hills and on interesting terrain that challenges you. You're wasted on pavement!

The Tip-toer

These runners look like their trainers are mini pogo sticks, springing along and having a ball with it. Every stride has a bouncy flourish and they're often ready with a big happy smile. They make running look such fun, you can't help but want to have a go.

If you're a Tip-toer, try: Honestly, just run anywhere and everywhere! Spread the running joy and get everyone doing it.

The 'All the Gear'

This running type has everything – the technical trainers, the hydration vest and the latest wearable tech to track all their stats. They look the part and *might* be pros, but is it a case of 'all the gear … no idea'? That has to be a case-by-case assessment, but either way, you can't fault their commitment to 'being a runner'.

If you're an 'All the Gear', try: Long urban routes, through places where you can see and be seen, with plenty of cool sights for selfie stops. If you can get some elevation in as well, that'll be interesting for your stats!

The School Run-ner

They're dressed for a run, head-to-toe in Lycra and checking their fitness tracker. They drop the kids at school, then off they go, but do they actually run afterwards? Maybe they're using the motivational trick of putting the kit on to show intent – and good luck to them, you've got this!

If you're a School Run-ner, try: Sticking to your intention. A lap round the school or a local park after drop-off, or maybe some hill sprints near where you've parked. Something quick you can fit in before work or whatever else you have planned for the day. Maybe treat yourself to a nice coffee afterwards – you did it, congratulate yourself!

The parkrunner

They *love* running, but mainly a 5K in the local park on a Saturday because they love running with lots of others. They might even collect the parkrun T-shirts and proudly wear them when occasionally running at other times. The parkrunner might not consider themselves a 'proper' runner but even if you only do that one run a week, you're still in the club.

If you're a parkrunner, try: Staying consistent with your parkrun, you're doing great! Want to run more? See if you can convince a few friends to do a 5K in a local park or just around where you live once a month, or even once a week. Keep it social, keep it fun, just keep running.

The Keeno

The Keeno runs everywhere. Everywhere they go, they talk about running. They do fifty-two races a year and all their social avatars are of them running. Every weekend, they are … yup, you guessed it, running. This is the borderline between hobby runner and pro, and honestly, I'm here for it!

If you're a Keeno, try: Joining a running club, so you can run even more, find brand new races and be with loads of people who love talking (and eating, sleeping and breathing) running just as much as you do!

OK, so this is by no means a serious analysis. It's my own personal observations and a bit of fun, but it makes a serious point: knowing how you run, why you run and what gives you your runner's high is so important. After all, you'll only stick with it if it makes you feel good. So, find your style, find your running joy and make running work for you.

SARA'S STORY

Sara Davies, MBE, is a very busy woman. A high-powered business executive, she's a mum, one of the Dragons on the BBC's *Dragons' Den* and a former contestant on *Strictly Come Dancing*. So how does she fit it all in? She lives by the same motto my family have teased me for using: If you want a job done, give it to a busy person.

When she came on *RunPod* in July 2023, Sara told me that she noticed how her efficiency improved once she started a family: 'Before I had kids, I could just work all the hours that God sent and then all of a sudden, once you have them, you have a reason why you want to shut your laptop at 5 o'clock and go home,' she said. 'But it's not acceptable to get less done in the day than I would have done, so you just have to get it all done to finish at 5 o'clock and it's amazing how much more efficient you become.'

This increased efficiency opened Sara's eyes to other ways she might maximise her schedule. 'If I can do that once, I can start to fit other things in,' she told me. 'Hence, when I did *Strictly*, I didn't stop anything else in my life – I still had the business, I still had the investment portfolio, I was still seeing the kids, doing the school runs and everything – and then all of a sudden, I managed to fit in forty hours of dancing a week as well!'

Of course, she didn't stop there and later decided

to squeeze running into her life too. Working to a strict schedule, with things like summer holidays planned months in advance, Sara shares a little printed schedule with her 'four amazing grandparents' – a support network she feels lucky and grateful to have – that they all use to co-ordinate holidays and activities around, and 'just make it work'. The reason for this is the value that Sara places on running in her life. She said: 'I am happier in my life when I am doing some running as well. I can't even explain why that is, I just feel like I am a better person.'

Like all of us, Sara had to find the best time to fit running into her particular schedule. 'I always do my running of a morning, it's the only time I can fit it in,' she explained. 'I had this lightbulb moment once when I realised that if I get up and go running on a morning, and then get show-ered and start my day and everything like that, I totally – no pun intended – hit the ground running. I'm into work at 8 o'clock and I am firing on all cylinders.

'If I compare that with a day when I haven't done that and I've dragged myself out of bed and I've just about got through the shower, it's been a hassle getting the kids off to school and I'm driving to work trying to psych myself up and I'll walk into work at 8 o'clock, thinking "oh God, here we go".'

The difference in her mental capacity on running and non-running days proved a game changer: 'People will always say to me, "But are you not tired from getting up an hour earlier or using all that energy on a morning?"' she said. 'And I'm like, "Well, I might be, but that is nothing compared to what I've got from it." The pay-off is negligible for what you get in return.'

It's not easy to stick to though, so how does she get up and out, even on days when she wants to curl back under the covers?

'For me, I need accountability. So now, for accountability, what I'll do is I'll say to my husband the night before, "I'm getting up early in the morning, sweetheart, cause I'm going for a run." I'll tell him and I'll put my running kit outside the bedroom door.

'My alarm goes off at 5.25 a.m., so I literally roll out of bed, step outside the door so I'm not disturbing him any longer than I need to and pull on my running gear before my mind has even engaged that it's twenty-five-past-bloody-five in the morning and I'd rather hit "snooze" and be in bed for another forty minutes, I just get out and go. And within ten minutes I'm fine.'

Sara Davies is a shining example of fitting running into your life no matter how busy you are. But she does it because of the value that running holds in her life, what it gives back to her – something I'm sure we can all relate to and definitely something we can learn from her. In her own words: 'Whatever goes on of a morning, I get up and run and I am a better person after it. I've never known something so good for you on so many levels.'

3

EXPLORING NEW PLACES

There's one benefit of running that isn't talked about enough – the freedom it gives you to explore. Not just places, but thoughts, ideas and experiences. Running really opens your eyes to wherever you happen to be doing it.

Now, when I started out, I picked a familiar route that I knew and was comfortable with, but that changed very quickly! I began adding distance, by running one street further along, taking a left instead of a right and exploring footpaths that branched out from my well-trodden route. Soon I discovered new ways to get to places that I would often go, shortcuts – and long ones when I wasn't quite ready to end my run – and a whole new world opened up to me. It gave me a new sense of my local geography:

where I was physically in relation to my home, work, friends' homes and favourite haunts. Being based in Southwest London and working in Central London, if I didn't run then I would get a car, a tube or a bus to and from work. I would stick to roads, all the major thoroughfares, and I would see the same things, day in and day out. That is, if I wasn't scrolling on my phone, as we all do.

Is it any wonder the average commute seems like such a slog?

Through running, where I go now varies from day to day. I've run past Buckingham Palace and down The Mall, soaking in the grandeur of the architecture; through Hyde Park in all the different seasons, noticing the different sounds, sights and smells; I've even run through Regent's Park and realised that you can see and hear all the animals in London Zoo – I actually got to run past the giraffes on my way home from work! The amazing bridges along the River Thames, the London Eye, Big Ben and Kensington Palace Gardens have all featured in my runs. I feel like a tourist in the place I live and commute all of the time. These days I never stop taking photos and I'm constantly seeing things in a brand-new light. This is where running stops being just physical and becomes an emotional and inspirational experience too.

RUNNER'S EXPLORATION

Exploring when you run isn't really something you decide to do, it just happens. Many of us start off so concerned that people are staring at us but we fail to realise that when we're out, no one is looking at us and we're not looking at other people either.

Our minds are far too busy taking in everything that's around us.

With running, you get to look up. You get to see things, you get to hear things, you get to smell things. I'll be honest, the latter isn't always a positive. Like in summer sometimes when you're running along, marvelling at how everything is stunning, the sun is warming your skin and then, BAM! A bin lorry drives past and all you can think is, *Oh, good grief, that stinks!* But more often than not, you'll notice the fragrance of the gorgeous flowers that have popped up in your local park, or between the cracks in the pavement, how different the air smells when you run just after rainfall, or when the weather warms, or even that there's a flock of birds living in the trees on your road that treat you to a dawn chorus every day.

The more I ran, the more things I noticed on my Botanic Gardens loop. The more I noticed, the more curious I became. I'd be almost home when I'd go, *I could turn right and go home here, but what if I went straight on, then turned right? Where would that take me?* Sometimes, it would just be a similar, but longer route back home but other times I'd spot a new shop, a pretty house or a pathway or green space I hadn't known existed.

When the Covid-19 pandemic took hold in 2020, lots of us really started exploring our own neighbourhoods through running, cycling and walking. With the restrictions that were in place, particularly when we were limited to one hour of outdoor exercise each day, it was really all anyone could do.

During that time, I remember running across Trafalgar Square and along The Mall in London. I was the only person running outside Buckingham Palace – in fact, I was the only person on the roads, full stop. There were no cars around at all – I also ran to Knightsbridge at one stage and I was literally running in the middle of the road, completely unthinkable in normal times.

As I went past Harrods, I looked up at the building. It was all lit up, but there wasn't another soul there. On a warm summer's day like that, it would usually have been heaving with tourists and there would be thousands of cars passing through, horns beeping and engines revving. But it was completely silent, apart from birds singing. I stopped and just stared in amazement. Admittedly, it felt a little freaky, like something out of the film *28 Days Later*, but it was quite special. A building in a place that was so familiar, like I'd never seen it before – I don't think I'll ever forget that experience.

On a less extreme level (and I don't think any of us want to experience that particular extreme again), this is the opportunity that running presents: a chance to see the places we know so well completely differently. You'll find that the adventurer in you becomes more intrepid as your confidence in running improves, but it always remains that you really don't have to go very far to explore.

NINE TIPS FOR EXPLORING LOCALLY

Running really is a fantastic way to explore your own local area, and there are some brilliant ways to see the places you go every day in a whole new light.

* Do your regular route the opposite way round: You'll see things from a different perspective doing your route backwards. But beware: the run will feel different too. That lovely downward slope you enjoy so much will be a hill in the opposite direction!

* Run into a park or gardens, not around them: If you usually run around a park or similar, why not venture inside, follow the paths and see what's there? You might find ponds, ornamental gardens or beautiful buildings to explore.

* Run up and down every street: Pick an area close to your home and run up and down every street within it.

You might find hidden pathways, a new shop or restaurant – or you can just have a peek at the houses.

✳ Find the highest point in your area: Run there, can you see your house? Either way, enjoy the descent home! One for the hill runners among you …

✳ Follow a feature of the local landscape: Is there a stream, river or canal nearby? A bridleway or footpath? Follow it and see where it takes you …

✳ Do your usual route at a different time of day: The sights, smells and sounds on your usual route will be completely different between morning, afternoon and evening. Why not try them all and compare?

✳ Run to a friend's house: Or anywhere you might usually drive or catch a bus to. If it's not too far, you can have a brew and run back. You never know what you might discover on the way.

✳ Follow a shape: You can use apps like Strava and MapMyRun to run a route that draws a shape on a map. At Christmas, where I live, local runners try to run the shape of a Christmas tree. It takes planning on a map but looks impressive when you post it to your socials!

✳ Follow another runner's route: Don't *actually* follow them, that would be creepy! But if you have friends who run locally, ask where they go, or check the routes that other runners have logged on Strava, MapMyRun or similar apps for inspiration.

FINDING YOUR FREEDOM

Exploring new things about familiar places is one thing, but the amazing thing about running is that it gives you the complete freedom to explore wherever you are. Whether it's a new town or city or a new country, as long as you have your kit, you're ready to go! If you want to try something new, and maybe a little more challenging, I recommend getting out to your nearest hills, countryside or coastline for some trail running. Trail running is perhaps most simply described as running in the heart of nature and we're lucky in the UK that nature is usually not much further than an hour or so from where we live.

With rugged paths, steep ascents and rolling descents, it's a world away from city running; think the Lake District, the Peak District, Dartmoor, Loch Lomond and the Brecon Beacons. It's a chance to really breathe in some clean, fresh air and expose yourself to incredible wildlife, views, landscapes and of course, the elements!

When it comes to travelling further afield, there are two types of people: those who take their sports kit and those who don't. I'm definitely the former – when I go away, the first thing to go in my case is my trainers. It was a bit of an evolution, though. I started out taking just one set of kit, but quickly realised that once used, it needed to be washed and I couldn't do that in time for my next run. So, I began taking two lots, then three … I think my case is now usually 80 per cent sports kit and 20 per cent dresses for evenings out!

Running gives you a great reason to get out, when you're away, beyond just keeping fit. The very first opportunity I have, when I arrive somewhere new, I get out and explore. I find it's the best way to get your bearings and really know where you are. As a morning runner, I love getting out early, but this holds even more benefits when you're abroad in popular holiday destinations.

The first thing is that you'll be up and about before the other tourists. You get to see a place slowly wake up and come to life, see where the locals go and get an unbiased opinion on what's there and what's good without having to work it out from among hordes of holidaymakers. You're not being swayed to where the popular parts of town are, you're just judging it for yourself, from what you can see in front of you. It also gives you the chance to see incredible landmarks that are usually overcrowded in all their glory.

I remember doing this in the beautiful Baroque island of Ortigia in Sicily, running through old parts of town and down the fortress walls of this city. The sun was shining, not too hot, but enough to warm your whole body, and with breathtaking views, it was stunning. There was hardly anyone else around, it was so peaceful – a world away from what it was like when I returned later in the day to the heaving crowds in the searing heat. I don't think I'd have liked to be the sweaty runner trying to get through them!

While my love of the morning recce does offer plenty of benefits for my husband, James, and daughter, Ella – I'll have found shortcuts and amazing hidden bakeries and restaurants before they've even woken up – they *do* have to put up with me boring them! We'll head out and they'll just be starting to find their feet, when I'll say: 'Oh by the way, you can turn right here. There's a path that goes all the way around there, it's really nice. There's a lovely bar at the end … blah, blah, blah.' I know they quite like it, but after an hour or so, they'll be begging me, 'Please don't tell us everywhere you've been running!'

Getting out for a run when I'm away for work is great too. Rather than getting in the car, being taken for filming, doing the job and coming back, I get to explore and form my own opinions of a place. To see it first-hand without a tour guide or a show script telling me what to think or say about a building, landmark or town. Learning that stuff later is better when it's enriching your own thoughts and experiences.

By the way, when you're running in new places, your routes don't have to be complex or challenging. Even a lap around the block gives you the chance to see, hear and smell all the things you'd miss in a car or bus. You can just get out there and soak up the ambiance, all within minutes of arriving. It's so easy!

If you're not quite ready for solo running in a foreign country or an unfamiliar town or city, and you fancy some sightseeing, you might want to try a running tour. It's just like city walking tours or using a tour guide except you run around all of the sights instead of walking. This is also great if you live in a big city and want to explore new areas. London has Secret London Runs, which has lots of themed runs, from trailblazing East End women to routes taking in the Christmas lights, while Birmingham has Run of a Kind Birmingham for exploring the city. For global locations, try RunningTours.net or Go Running Tours (the latter also cover the fantastic city of Edinburgh, if you fancy a running tour there).

Regardless of whether I plan to run alone or with others, when I travel somewhere new, I will always do a bit of an online recce first. This is not just to find places that might be enjoyable to run, like a beach, the seafront, park, a local trail or past interesting landmarks, but to make sure I know where it is safe.

STAYING SAFE

As fantastic as exploring places – new or familiar – is, it's important to always keep your safety in mind. There have been places I have travelled, like Brazil, where I have been advised not to run. At home as well, there are places and times that I won't run. I run in the morning, or during daylight hours, not just because it suits my schedule, but also because it's when I feel safest.

Years ago, I remember walking through the Botanic Gardens in Glasgow at dusk. I felt scared and vulnerable, and I haven't forgotten that feeling. There are, unfortunately, many reasons why people – particularly women – don't feel safe when running. In fact, in the National Women's Running Survey of 2022[3], 18 per cent of respondents said that they had considered stopping running altogether due to safety concerns.

Now, for the men reading this book, this isn't your cue to stop reading and skip to the next section. Staying safe when running is important and relevant to people of any gender, and much of the advice is the same for all of us. But even where the advice and experiences are specific to women runners, it's important that men understand them too. As runners, we're a community and we all have to look out for one another.

By the time I'd established myself as 'someone who runs' and was running from work after my morning show, people would assume that I ran in as well. When I'd appear in the studio in my kit, ready for my run home, people would ask: 'Oh, have you run in?' to which I'd respond, 'Not a chance in hell' – I'd got a taxi in, of course. My day started at 4.30 a.m. In autumn and winter, it would still be pitch-black when I arrived at work, let alone when I set off. Now, I'm sure that some people do enjoy running at night, but it's not for me, or pretty much any woman that I know.

When Samsung released an advert in 2022, showing a woman running through a city at 2 a.m., with headphones on, it received a huge public backlash and also prompted discussion in the *RunPod* Facebook group. The consensus was clear: it was unrealistic. Women don't run at night because they are scared to – and with good reason. The National Women's Running Survey 2022 revealed that 47 per cent of respondents had been verbally harassed and 11 per cent had been followed or intimidated while running, and there have been many recent and high-profile cases of women being physically harassed or assaulted while out running. It really doesn't matter how confident or experienced you are, there are always risks. But that doesn't mean we have to stop. In fact, we absolutely should not. It just means that it's important to be aware of the dangers and protect yourself against them.

RUNNING SAFETY ESSENTIALS FOR EVERYONE

As with all things, it's important to take safety into consideration. Making decisions based on where you will be running, at what time and the conditions you will be running in will ensure you're well-prepared for any eventuality and can really enjoy your run.

* Run in daylight – If this isn't possible, stick to well-lit routes, or consider using a treadmill in the gym instead.

* Make sure there are other people around – Run in a group, or if you can't or don't want to do that, run where there are others. You could even tail another group of runners, so there's people around should anything happen.

* Take your phone with you – You can call for help if needed or use Google Maps if you're lost. Also, make sure you add your ICE – 'In Case of Emergency' – contact to your address book as this is what emergency services will look for if they need to contact friends or family on your behalf.

* Let people know where you're going, and when you'll be back – Put a Post-it on the fridge, send a simple text to a friend, or even share your live location in WhatsApp or Strava.

* Take local advice – If you're running abroad, plan ahead and check if it's safe to run there. When you arrive, ask hotel staff or a local information centre if there are places and times you should avoid running.

* Stay aware – If you want to listen to music, keep it low so you can still hear oncoming traffic and be aware of what and who is around you. You could even try bone conduction headphones. These work by transmitting sound vibrations along your cheekbones instead of through the air, so you can listen to music while still hearing surrounding noise.

* Wear reflective clothing – If you're running at night or in low-light conditions, this can help drivers see you on the road.

* Face oncoming traffic – Where possible, run on the side of the road facing the oncoming traffic, particularly if you're running in the countryside.

* Keep something in the tank – Don't run until you're flat out, hold something back in case you do need to run away in an emergency.

* Trust your gut – If something doesn't feel right, it possibly isn't. Trust your instincts and get yourself to a safe place if you feel anything is off.

ADVICE FOR THE GUYS

When Mayor of London Sadiq Khan came on *RunPod*, he said it best when he told me: 'I've got to recognise that my experiences are very different to yours.' Running *is* a different experience for women and one of the most important things that male runners can do to support female runners is to understand those differences and be aware of their behaviour.

'It starts with unhealthy attitudes, unhealthy comments, that leads to unhealthy behaviour that affects women's safety,' Sadiq continued. 'Whether it's safe enough or not [to run] is a secondary issue. The fact that women don't feel it's safe is a problem for me.'

There are lots of things that you can do as a male runner to make women feel safer when you're out running, day or night:

* Keep your distance – If you find yourself jogging or running behind a woman, pause to give her some space or cross the road so you aren't behind her any more.

* Be respectful – By all means smile and greet women runners, but don't make inappropriate comments, even if you think it's a compliment. If they don't engage, don't push it – just carry on with your run.

* Read body language – Be aware if you are making a woman uncomfortable. Things like slowing down/

speeding up, turning her body away from you or avoiding eye contact are all signs to end the conversation and leave her alone.

* Don't sneak up – If you need to pass a woman while running, a friendly 'passing on your right/left' while you're still a distance away can be a welcome heads-up. Give her lots of room too, don't brush right by her.

* Don't be offended – Women's wariness is natural. They have no way of knowing you're not a threat, so don't take it personally.

* Call out disrespectful comments – If you see other men, particularly friends and family, making disrespectful comments to women runners, or engaging in any behaviours that may make them feel uncomfortable, challenge them and explain why it's not acceptable.

* Listen to women runners – Be a part of your community, listen to the experiences of women runners and always be willing to learn, so you can help make running safer for them.

* Share these tips – Help make running safer for women by sharing these simple tips with people you know.

GETTING LOST IN A GOOD RUN

When you're out on a run, it's the perfect time to let your mind wander too. Away from all the bustle of your day-to-day life, you can explore new ideas, creative projects, or even plan your week ahead. The time you give to yourself when you run is just that – yours. You should use it to your advantage, whether that's creatively or practically.

I've lost count of the ideas that have come to me when I've been running home and that I've been able to nurture and develop just because there's nothing else that I need to be doing at that moment. The mind space gives me clarity and the chance to think about what might be possible. It really gets the creative juices flowing!

I also love to multitask and I see running as an opportunity to listen to a podcast or some music and go through upcoming plans in a way that I can't when I'm at work or looking after my family. I'll find myself having to stop to write a note in a moment of inspiration, email to arrange an appointment or make a quick phone call when I remember something important. It helps me to get things done. And let me tell you, you can get a lot done too! I ran the London Marathon in 2010, just over a month before my wedding. I put my headphones on, with a playlist packed with Kings of Leon, The Killers, Keane and Lady Gaga, and just started planning.

Details for the florist, bridesmaid duties, seating plan …

After three hours and thirty-one minutes focused on the task, I had everything boxed off. It was brilliant, completely effective and left me with loads more time to celebrate my new PB with a nice cocktail at the end!

Letting your mind run free when you're out can be a chance to cleanse the mind too. If something has been stressing me out, or there's a problem that I've been struggling to find a solution to, I also know that I'll be able to work through it as I pound along the pavements. By the time I'm home, I feel happier, lighter and more able to manage difficult situations. It's a mental freedom that I've come to really appreciate over the years.

GETTING LOST ON A GOOD RUN

Now, getting lost in your own mind on a run is excellent and I highly recommend it. Getting lost while on a good run is a whole other matter and something that I know lots of people worry about, particularly in new and unfamiliar places. My very first guest on *RunPod*, back in March 2019, was the pop and TV star, Peter Andre. During our chat he admitted that getting lost is the only thing he has difficulty with when running in new places, often having to ring someone to find and collect him, based just on what he can see around him.

I've also been lost a good few times and I'm always eternally grateful for GPS to help me navigate home. It can be a bit scary if you find yourself unsure of where you are and it's easy enough to do, but there are a few things you can do to give yourself a helping hand and some confidence while you're out.

You can map your planned route on an app like MapMyRun, which covers fourteen countries globally, including the UK, the United States, Australia, New Zealand, Spain and Japan, and take your phone with you so you can navigate back if you get lost (it also has lots of local running routes you can follow as well).

If you're somewhere completely new, maybe run a straight 'there and back' route to a significant location, like a tourist attraction or a park, so there's no twists and turns to be confused by. If that's not possible, just be sure to make a mental note of any landmarks or distinctive buildings or natural features that will help you find your way back.

If you do find yourself totally lost, it's OK to get a little help. Always having some cash, your bank card or your phone with you means you can jump in a cab or on public transport if need be.

A really useful app to have on your phone is What-3Words[4]. The developers have divided the entire globe into 57 trillion 3 x 3m squares and assigned each one a unique combination of three words, which can be shared with emergency services so they can pinpoint where you are. It even works offline, so it's ideal if you're somewhere remote, or with poor signal, like in the hills, near the sea or in the countryside.

As you build your confidence in running, you'll find it easier to get out and explore. You might even end up like me and go from wandering just a little further off your usual route each time to booking your holidays based solely on where you fancy running.

After years of turning up at our resort only to find that we are conveniently right next to a dream running route, I think my family have finally cottoned on. I'm sure it drives them mad, but I make no apologies! I've used running to explore Glasgow and London – my hometown and the place I now call home – and around the UK and the rest of the world, from Eastbourne to East Lothian, Cape Town to Cape Wrath, New York City to Washington, D.C., and so many more amazing places. As incredible as all of these adventures have been, though, none compare to that of one of my favourite *RunPod* guests, whose experience can only be described as out-of-this-world …

NICK'S STORY

Taking exploring new places with running to a whole other level, in 2019 Nick Butter became the first man to run a marathon in every country in the world, 194 in total – wow!

Nick took on the challenge to raise money for Prostate Cancer UK, and when he joined me on *RunPod* for a post trip debrief in January 2020, he'd raised almost £200,000.

The first country on his itinerary was Canada, where Nick ran in freezing -25-degree conditions in Toronto on 6 January 2018. Extreme conditions were a theme throughout the trip, with thunderstorms in Hong Kong, blistering heat in Brunei, smog and dust in Madagascar and a top temperature of 59 degrees in Kuwait.

He also had to navigate difficult terrain, like the mountains in Nepal and Bolivia, sudden changes in conditions from country to country, and a punishing schedule. Nick told me: 'I was flying from Bolivia all the way over to North Korea and then back to Ecuador. One minute I was running in snow in Pyongyang and then five days later I was running back at the equator in Ecuador.'

It wasn't just the incredible places that Nick experienced that made his journey, it was the people he met too. He said: 'I didn't really know what to expect when travelling around the world and doing all this running. I was doing three marathons a week, every week for ninety-six weeks, but every single step of the way I had people who were totally and utterly selfless and they came out and supported me.'

When his challenge was complete Nick counted up the new contacts in his phone – the people he had spent substantial time with and now called his friends. There were 2,411 of them, all spread around the globe and many with whom he had stayed. He said: 'I was hosted by many, many brilliant families. Frequently, none of them spoke a word of English and that would then force me to learn different languages or at least try and understand and eventually learn.'

When I asked Nick where he'd enjoyed running the most, he shared his love of Sierra Leone and its people and of running around a beautiful volcano in the city of Antigua Guatemala, but spoiled for choice, he had to pick a whole *continent* as his favourite place to run – South America.

His reason for running was more definitive. He told me: 'A lot of people see the world through social media or TV. But if you're running you see the world through your own eyes. You meet people and it's a great way to connect, but you always come back with a sense of feeling better. Whether it's happier, whether it's stronger or more out-of-breath, or just being set free and exploring the world with your two feet.'

What a perfect way to see the world from a completely different perspective!

TOP TEN UK CITIES TO RUN IN

Completing a marathon in every country in the world is something few of us are ever likely to be able to do, but there are still lots of places to explore closer to home. If you're seeking inspiration, look no further – with the help of *RunPod* listeners, I've compiled the top ten UK cities to run. So, find your freedom and get exploring!

1. London – This city really has everything – grand parks, historic landmarks, built-up urban areas, paths along the River Thames … I could go on forever. Five of its major parks are also relatively interconnected – Hyde Park, Kensington Gardens, Green Park, St James's Park and Regent's Park – so there's hours of exploring there alone!

2. Glasgow – As a Glaswegian myself, I might be biased, but you really are spoilt for choice for running spots in and out of the city. There are flat roads and steep inclines in the city centre, there's a lovely riverside area by the Clyde and a ton of beautiful parks to explore. You can also jump in a car and head a few miles outside town to explore coastline, lochs and the Campsie Fells.

3. Brighton – There are more than ten miles of seafront paths in Brighton, as well as a gorgeous trail running in the countryside near the city. For a slightly more

challenging run, head to South Downs National Park, where there are rolling hill trails running through a stunning mixture of open countryside and woodland.

4. Edinburgh – Beautiful, historic and hilly – very hilly! Edinburgh's inclines can seem a bit intimidating, but with the majority of its famous landmarks and architectural highlights all within around a 4–5-mile journey, running them is a great way of soaking up the sights. If you're brave and fancy a challenge, you can always run up Arthur's Seat – a big, gradual 2.4-mile hill, it's classified as moderate to difficult, making it accessible to most runners.

5. Leeds – There are some excellent loops through Leeds city centre, as well as fantastic runs along the canals, to keep you entertained. Whether you're after a short jog around Burley Park or a half-marathon route that circles the whole city, there are options for all skill levels to enjoy without having to travel too far from the centre.

6. Cambridge – A beautiful running location, with extensive paths along the River Cam and large greens close to the city centre. You can run around the campus at the University of Cambridge or, if you're feeling fancy, the English Country Estate at Wimpole Hall.

7. York – A small city, steeped in Roman history and packed with great running routes. There's a wonderful 3-mile loop along the ancient city walls. I recommend running along the perimeter starting near the Treasurer's House, but if you want to go off-piste, you can also take a loop around the Yorkshire Museum Gardens and breathe in the botanicals or run along the banks of the River Ouse.

8. Truro – Truro's narrow streets have a great buzz. You can run to the city's gorgeous cathedral, up to Victoria Gardens while seeing the sights on the way. Then, from Victoria Gardens, you can add a mile to your route by doing a loop there. If you don't fancy running in town, you can run along the River Truro to Malpas – but maybe one for a drier day as the dirt path can get a bit muddy!

9. Cardiff – The favourite choice for running in the Welsh capital is the chain of parks and multi-use paths along the River Taff. Try the popular 6-kilometre route starting in Bute Park, northwest of the city centre. Run along the Dock Feeder Canal and the Blackweir Fields, then run northwest towards Cardiff University. Cross the river and head back along the River Taff trail and Pontcanna Fields. Or what about the Cardiff Bay Trail? Ten kilometres of great views from beaches, bridges and wetlands.

10. Inverness – A city that holds a special place in my heart because I carried the Olympic torch into the heart of it, back in 2012 – what an honour! It's also home to the Inverness Grand Tour, a walking and running route starting in the centre at the Great Glen Way path on the east side of the River Ness, near Bellefield Park. Cross the small bridge to Ness Islands to a tree-lined walking path and go half a mile, crossing over the west bank and run through Whin/Canal Park, continuing to the Botanical Gardens, Inverness Leisure Centre with its own running track and then continue to Bught Park Pitches, finishing off with a 1-mile River Ness Loop to Ness Bridge, passing Inverness Castle – stunning!

4

THE INEXPLICABLE JOY
OF A GOOD RUN

Like lots of runners, I love the way running makes me *feel*. Not just that runner's high that we all chase – that's the pinnacle of course, the holy grail – but the sensation on every step along the way. We all experience it differently, but most would agree that it's a feeling of joy that courses through your whole body, radiates energy and can change how you feel for the rest of the day. To be honest, it's pretty inexplicable, but I'm going to try my best to explain here how it feels for me.

I'm always excited to run, so I'm buzzing even before I start, anticipating all the benefits I'm going to get from my run. No matter how I feel beforehand, I know I will feel better afterwards and that's worth getting excited about. Once I start, I'm aware of how my body feels, feet pounding the pavements, arms swinging alternately to my stride, getting into tempo with my quickening pulse as my heart starts pumping blood to my muscles and brain. For the first five to ten minutes, my breathing is heavy, my throat burns and I can feel my cheeks getting flushed. This is always the toughest part of any run, but I keep going because I know what's coming. Then, my head clears and suddenly the running doesn't feel so tough anymore. I feel good – no, actually, I feel AMAZING! I'm glowing with sweat, beaming with joy and loving every second.

It's happened – I've hit my stride and the endorphins are finally flowing.

At this point, I forget any aches and pains – temporarily at least – as I'm carried through the rest of my run on a wave of feelgood hormones. By the time I'm done, the serotonin's pumping and all the endorphins are going crazy in my body. Am I tired and sweaty? Yes, of course! But I'm also energised, I'm invigorated, I'm clear-headed and I feel so good in a way that I really can't explain. I feel completely euphoric. I've got it, I've got my runner's high! Now, that feeling can stay with me for the whole of the day, it really is something special. But what is it that causes a runner's high?

THE SCIENCE BEHIND THE 'RUNNER'S HIGH'

Before we get into what causes the 'runner's high' and makes us feel so amazing that we can't help coming back for more, what actually is a 'runner's high'? In its simplest form it's a feeling of elation brought on by continuous aerobic exercise. It can differ in its intensity and effects from person to person, but often includes a feeling of exhilaration, calm or positivity, as well as reduced awareness of pain and discomfort, and lower stress levels – all combining to give us that sensation of being 'high'. This is known as a 'neurobiological effect' of physical exercise, the way that exercise can change your mind state. Any form of moderately strenuous exercise can cause this response, but running is particularly good for providing the conditions needed to elicit these responses in the body.

For a long time, one of our body's 'feelgood' or 'happy' hormones, endorphins, has been credited with delivering our runner's high, but there's actually more to it than that. To understand it better, let's break down what actually happens in our body when we run[5].

1. Hormone Hero #1: Acetylcholine
Five to ten minutes into your run.
OK, so not technically a hormone hero for running, but when you start running, acetylcholine (ACh) is busy doing

its job of looking after your body in its resting state; dilating your blood vessels, slowing your heart rate down and other functions that promote relaxation. However, it's the exact opposite of what you need on a run. So, when your body detects 'stress' as you start running, it calls on the body to 'fight' it, getting rid of acetylcholine and creating the hormones that you need in your new state (more on them in a moment).

This transition is why the start is undeniably the hardest part of any run as your body shifts from a resting state into an aerobic state and you need more oxygen delivered to your muscles. Your heart is basically trying to catch up with the demand, which is why you're out of puff and your heart is racing when you first get going.

You're not unfit – it's science!

2. Hormone Hero #2: Endorphins

Released twenty to thirty minutes into a run.

There's a reason why people equate the sensation of a 'runner's high' to being high on drugs – endorphins are in fact opiates that your body produces naturally in the central nervous system and pituitary gland. They are released during exercise, as well as in response to pleasurable activities like eating or sex. Once released, they are sensed by the brain's prefrontal and limbic regions: the former is responsible for the control and organisation of your emotional reactions, while the latter works to make you feel good, avoid pain and generally does the job of keeping you alive.

Now, this is important. The runner's high doesn't just exist for our enjoyment (rude, I know!). Endorphins are also released as a reaction to pain and discomfort, to reduce those feelings and allow the body to keep functioning. This would have been very useful for our ancestors, who had to spend long days hunting in extreme conditions, perhaps with fatigue, injury or having not eaten for a while. Scientists believe that what we call 'runner's high' might actually have developed to get us through long periods of running and hunting, numbing pain and ensuring our survival. Think about that next time you're out for your run!

As those parts of your brain sense your endorphins, they light up. The more you push yourself on your run, the more endorphins rush to the brain. The more endorphins the brain senses, the stronger that euphoric feeling gets – incredible!

While endorphins are what we've all been trained to chase, more recent research[6] has revealed there is a bit more to it and endorphins can't actually do the job on their own. Why? Well, it turns out they're too big to pass through the blood-brain barrier on their own. If they can't do that, then they can't change your brain state. They need another hormone, endocannabinoids, which are small enough to cross the blood-brain barrier, to help them along.

3. Hormone Hero #3: Endocannabinoids

Released twenty to thirty minutes into a run.

Now, research into endocannabinoids (the body's natural form of THC, the most active compound in cannabis) and exercise is still quite limited, but a type of endocannabinoid called anandamide has been found at high levels in the blood of people who've recently completed a run.

The endocannabinoid system hormones are believed to have a very important regulatory role in the secretion of hormones related to reproductive functions and response to stress, the latter being pertinent to running. Not only are endocannabinoids small enough to cross the blood-brain barrier, but they can also be made by almost any cell in the body (unlike endorphins, which can only be created by specific neurons), so there's a much bigger potential for them to have an impact on your brain state, making you feel elated, reducing anxiety and bringing a feeling of calm.

4. Hormone Hero #4: Serotonin

Released two to four hours after a run.

Another 'happy' hormone, serotonin is also a neurotransmitter, which means it sends chemical messages between the brain and body, telling it how to work. It primarily supports the function of relaxation and controlling your mood and happiness, as well as regulating sleep.

Exercise and spending time outside in the sunlight prompts the release of serotonin into the bloodstream, which is why runners often benefit from it. When your serotonin is at normal levels, you will feel calm, more focused and happier. A lack of serotonin is connected to issues such as depression and anxiety.

Unlike endorphins and endocannabinoids, the impact of serotonin only kicks in after exercise, usually two to four hours afterwards, when it is released along with other neurotransmitters, including norepinephrine, which improves attention levels and focus, and 'reward' chemical, dopamine, which is what provides you with that amazing sense of satisfaction from exercise.

HAVE I HAD A RUNNER'S HIGH?

Now, maybe you do a fifteen-minute jog three times a week and have been feeling great. But learning more about the science, you're now wondering if you've run for long enough for those fabulous endorphins to be released. Or maybe you don't quite connect to the feelings of complete elation described by others (or by the science).

If you look at the scientific definitions of a runner's high, what hormones are released and when, and what that should feel like, you might be asking yourself – have I experienced a runner's high at all? If you are, I have some questions for you. When you run, do you feel good? Do you feel happy? After your run, do you feel better than you did before?

If you answered yes to any of these questions, then I believe you've experienced a runner's high – your own runner's high. It might not align exactly with the scientific definition, but it's yours and it's unique. We all experience this inexplicable joy of running differently and our highs may vary in effects and intensity, but they're all real and valid – so just enjoy whatever form it takes.

For some people that high will come from just getting out the door and putting one foot in front of the other for as long as they are able or taking twenty minutes in the morning to get themselves in a good frame of mind for the day ahead. For others it will be a specific mile, or time into a race, when those endorphins start firing off, or at the end of a big race, with your family and friends cheering you over the finish line. My own runner's high has always come from that feeling of achievement, when the run is complete and I can say 'I did it'. That's as true for returning home after my commute run from work as it is for finishing the London Marathon – but that's just me!

RUNNING FOR YOUR MENTAL HEALTH

The way that running makes you feel isn't all about your hormones, it's the benefits you feel that are beyond that buzz and the physical impact of running for fitness. Although it might feel like it, the link between running and improved mental health isn't a new concept. The connection between regular running and positive mood changes, increased self-esteem and decreased anxiety have been discussed in research since 1979. But it wasn't really a common topic outside of academia until much more recently. Now, you can't move for people celebrating running's mental health benefits and the research supports it too.

In 2020, a large review of literature on the relationship between running and mental health was published by researchers, the first time in thirty years such an overview had been published. Across three main categories of running, all resulted in improved mental health[7]. And by the way, running has always helped my mental health, I just wouldn't have said that I ran for that reason back when I first started – it wasn't really something anyone discussed. I definitely recognise it now though.

Living between Leeds and Glasgow in my late teens and early twenties, with a relentless work schedule, I'd get upset that I wasn't with my best friends for special occasions, or that I couldn't go to family parties because I was away and had made commitments for work. Occasionally it would get me down, but then I'd go for a run. I'd start feeling tied up in knots with frustration about missing out on making memories, and worrying about letting family and friends down. Then, when out running, it was amazing to discover how that boost of serotonin and rush of endorphins brought so much clarity. It gave me an opportunity to mull things over with a more balanced perspective. Yes I might miss out on some important events but I was lucky to be doing a brilliant job that I loved, with amazing colleagues – this was what I had dreamt of. I always say that running simply gave me the chance to 'see the light'. It helped me see the positives of my situation too. At the time, I was single and all my friends had boyfriends or girlfriends. Saturday night always seemed to be date night, so I'd quite often spend it on my own rather than being out with my friends and sometimes it felt a bit rubbish. But, on Sunday morning, I'd be hangover-free and up early, out having a lovely run, feeling alive and refreshed. I realised then that there were advantages to being on my own on the weekend.

Without those runs I'd have felt anxious and lonely, isolated in my flat. At the time I saw them as doing what I could to look after myself, but I recognise now that what I was actually doing was using running to manage my mental health. Now, everyone who knows me knows that I'm an anxious person. I live by a schedule and I need to know what I'm doing, hour by hour, every day, or the stress creeps in. If I find myself slipping behind schedule, I'll start to panic and suddenly, I feel like I'm not in control anymore and all the things I thought it was possible to achieve start to slip away. The panic paralyses me and I can't think straight or find solutions in the way I usually would. My whole mind fills with angst and I'll spiral into a pit of negativity that drags me into a rut that I'll struggle to get out of.

The worst times of my life have been in those ruts but running absolutely eliminates them. As my feet hit the pavement I break through the worry and fear that has frozen me into inaction and I unravel it all in my head. I can see more clearly; I can organise things, I can find solutions. It never goes away, I know I will always have anxiety and stress, but I manage it by running. Rather than going straight from work to family commitments to bed and back round again the next day, it gives me time out of the game – some 'me' time to put everything into perspective. By doing this, I feel better and I don't bring it home to Ella or James. A simple run can completely change my outlook and how the world feels, and that's a very powerful thing!

That said, it's important to recognise that while running can certainly support your mental health, boosting your mood, relieving stress and even improving your sleep, it can't cure mental health problems alone. Mental health is part of our overall health and running can play a part in maintaining it, as it does our physical health. But you wouldn't run to cure a physical ailment, would you? You'd go to a doctor. The same should be true of mental health.

If you're struggling with a mental health issue or illness, reach out and get appropriate support. The Hub of Hope is a free website and app managed by mental health charity, Chasing the Stigma, that is a huge directory of local and national places to get help. There are currently more than 13,000 mental health support services across the UK listed and the app has a 'Need Help Now' function that allows you to talk directly to the Samaritans or access text message support via Shout by texting 85258.

BRYONY'S STORY

Author, journalist and podcaster Bryony Gordon first got into running in 2016 at a low point in her life. Having a history of depression, obsessive compulsive disorder (OCD), alcoholism and addiction, Bryony shared how she'd tried everything to make herself feel better when she joined me on *RunPod* in June 2020.

'I'd tried antidepressants, different quantities of alcohol and drugs, which let me tell you, don't work,' she said. 'I'd done therapy, I'd done everything, and I was like, "I think I am going to have to do this exercise thing that people are talking about, that they say is very good for your mental health."' So off she went, in leopard-print Converse trainers (just like me with my beginner fashion trainers) with a hole in the heel, her husband's tracksuit bottoms, *Star Wars* T-shirt and carrying water in her daughter's Tommee Tippee cup.

Bryony's book, *Mad Girl*, about her OCD, came out the same year she took up running, and she became involved in the royal mental health charity Heads Together, which had been announced as the official charity of the 2017 London Marathon.

Bryony said, 'Two thousand and seventeen was an absolutely huge year for me. I got offered a place for the marathon and I signed up, then I asked Prince Harry if he'd be the first guest on my mental health podcast, *Mad World*, and he said yes'.

A couple of months after the Marathon, Bryony got sober.

'I think the running had made me realise there was another way I could live than the way I was,' she revealed. 'Running genuinely has changed my life, I can't underestimate that. And it doesn't mean that I'm this squeaky-clean, green juice [person], I'm not. I'm still a size 18, I have my vices. I'm not perfect, and I've never claimed to be, and I make mistakes the whole time. But I keep going and running has allowed me to do that.

'I remember during my first marathon at mile twenty-one thinking, *this is so hard, is there ever going to be a time when I'm not running this marathon?* And then I remember thinking, *hang on, Bryony, you've been through way worse than this, you've had terrible depressions, you've had breakdowns and here, there are people cheering you on from the side of the road and giving you Haribo, just get on with it. This is not the worst thing you've ever been through.*

'Every time I think I can't do something, I remind myself I can do hard things. We can all do hard things; humans are remarkable and running reminds me of that.

'It reminds me that if I put in a training plan every week, my body can do something I didn't think it could the week before and that is just a remarkable feeling for someone with a history of bulimia and addiction and all of that stuff. It's putting faith in your body instead of having fear in it.'

While out running, Bryony listens to meditations on the free meditation app, Insight Timer, or the GABA podcast, using the time to further support her mental health.

'I find it's a real moment just to get out all the stresses and strains, all your fears for the day,' she said. 'They're inspiring. They're not meditation as you think a meditation would be.'

Bryony usually gets her runner's high at about mile eleven, but what does that feel like for her?

'It makes me feel like, oh my god, I can make this feeling with my own body. I have not had to go to the pub to do it,' she said.

That'll be the good old endorphins! Before we finished our chat, Bryony left me with some brilliant words of advice for anyone keen to start running: 'Keep going, do it for your head and for your heart and not for anything else, have a plan and stick to it and just enjoy yourself,' she said. 'And at the end, celebrate. Celebrate how bloody awesome you are because you've gone out and done that session and you are an absolute LEGEND!'

FROM COUCH TO RUNNER'S HIGH IN TEN MINUTES

The true beauty of running is just how easily accessible this truly amazing feeling is. You can be sitting on your couch one minute, decide you're going for a run and ten minutes later, you're out there and that buzz is kicking in. Unlike other workouts, you don't have to drive to a gym or swimming pool, book a tennis court or get to a golf course and it costs little to nothing to do. You just step outside (or onto your treadmill, if you have one at home) and you're off! Push past those tough first few minutes and you're up and away – instant high!

As I mentioned before, a good run feels different for everyone and no one's experience of a runner's high is the same. There is no 'right' way to achieve or experience a runner's high, but there are a few things you can do to increase the chances of those highs (or just boost whatever high your run gives you):

Push yourself, but not too hard – Endorphins and endocannabinoids are produced in response to stress, so a nice easy jog might not quite wake them up. You'll need to push yourself hard enough to feel the strain, but not so hard that you exhaust or injure yourself.

Run for longer periods – It typically takes about twenty to thirty minutes for endorphins to be released, so run for at least forty-five minutes to really feel that high.

Be consistent – If you're a relatively new runner, then running for forty-five minutes or more might not be possible at first. But if you run consistently, you will build up your stamina and endurance and you'll get there – and get that high!

Introduce other mood-boosters – Science tells us that we get serotonin from being out in the sunlight, so get yourself outside! Other research has found that people who undertake strenuous exercise together get a bigger rush of endorphins[8] and that listening to music we love can boost the release of dopamine and increase those happy chemical feelings[9].

BOOST THAT MOTIVATION

Despite knowing just how GREAT you will feel after your run, it can sometimes still be hard to find the motivation to get out there in the first place. Maybe you're feeling sluggish and tired, the rain outside is torrential or you just can't be bothered to go. Whatever the reason, it happens to all of us. I always think it would be great if you could bottle the way you feel, so when you're having one of those 'I can't be bothered' days, you could go to that bottle and remember what you'll get from it – instant motivation. It's not quite bottled, but I have found a way to do this that works for me and it might work for you too. At the end of a run, when you're feeling amazing, take a selfie.

OK, you might feel a bit silly taking a photo of yourself and you might look like a sweaty mess, but as you well know, you feel SO GOOD that you don't care! Just take the selfie – you don't have to put it anywhere, it's just for you – and save it to your phone. When you feel like you're not up for a run, all you have to do is go back to that photo, look at it and see how happy you were. Remember, *that's* how you're going to feel in ten, twenty, thirty minutes' time.

Now get out there and *feel* that run!

5

RAMPING UP
YOUR RUNNING

It's hard to pinpoint exactly when it happens, but for most people who get into running, there comes a moment when you go from being 'someone who runs' to 'being a runner'. It's quite subtle at first – looking for more opportunities to run, maybe taking your kit on holiday. You might find yourself thinking more about your times and distances or craning your neck while you're out to check out another runner's trainers or some other cool kit. Oh, and you'll want to talk about running *all the time*. This is the perfect time to start ramping up your running. You see, you know you can do it now. You know you enjoy it. So, what next?

Now, when I first started out, I quickly realised that running was my thing, but I would still never call myself a runner. 'Runners' were the Lycra-clad masses at the London Marathon start line; the professionals, loaded with gels and hydration packs and all checking their fitness watches. Then, when they set off, WOW! The skill, the pace … and then twenty miles later, looking like they'd barely broken a sweat.

I was someone who ran, *they* were runners.

Of course, I know now that runners from all walks of life take on marathons – I was literally watching the elites and wondering why I couldn't run like Paula Radcliffe. Not all of them wear Lycra – some come dressed as rhinos, skeletons and Big Ben. In fact, you don't even *have* to do races to be a runner.

It took about a year before I finally noticed the shift. Without thinking, I was taking my running kit away with me on holiday and for work travel. I'd see a really long straight road and instantly think, *I wonder how long it takes to run along that?*. I began to view my world through the prism of opportunities to run.

At the time my parents were still living down south, so I would go to visit them and catch up with old school friends while I was home. One friend lived eight miles away. Where in the past, I would have got in the car to go round, now I'd run to her house, have a cup of tea and a chat, then after an hour, run right back.

My parents would roll their eyes and say: 'Oh, she's off running again.'

Running rather than driving to visit friends became a habit. It just suddenly made so much sense to me – I was going to hang out with friends for a couple of hours and then I was going to come home. Why not couple that with some exercise? I knew I was a runner when I started doing stuff like that. The truth was I blooming loved it and realised how much I needed it in my life. I didn't run all that far, I wasn't fast and I wasn't great at it – but I was a runner. I guess this is where the obsession truly began. If you're feeling the same, there are some things that you might want to consider as you move from being a beginner into an intermediate runner.

UPGRADE YOUR KIT

The beauty of running is that you don't need any specialist kit but that's not to say you might not want it once you've really caught the running bug! As I've said before, branded and expensive items don't necessarily equal the best, but if you really have got into your running, you may want to invest a little more in branded running clothes and kit from specialist brands. If it makes your run better, more comfortable, or you just feel great in it, then it's worth the extra cost.

As well as an ever-expanding running wardrobe with shorts, leggings and tops for every possible occasion, there's a few other areas you might want to look at upgrading.

Trainers

As soon as you start running regularly, a couple of times a week or more, it's well worth investing in your trainers. While the exact mileage will depend on your weight and the terrain you run on, it's generally recommended that you replace running shoes every 300–500 miles – if you run about three miles, three times a week, this would be like getting a new pair around once a year. Investing in your running footwear isn't just financial – the best trainers for you won't necessarily be the most expensive pair anyway – but you might also need to invest a bit more time to find them.

I'd highly recommend visiting a specialist running shop to have your gait analysis done. It sounds super technical, but a simple way of looking at gait analysis is that it is the process of looking at how your feet hit the ground when you run.

Your 'gait' is your running stride – the movements your feet and legs make when you run. It will affect how and where your feet strike the floor – known as 'pronation' – and how it distributes the impact and absorbs the shock.

There are three types of gait:

Overpronation – When the foot rolls inward excessively. This can cause shin splints and lower back pain, among other conditions. It's the most common gait and is often seen in runners with flat feet or low arches.

Under pronation (supination) – When the foot doesn't roll inward very far, but instead rolls outward, putting pressure on the ankle and toes. Common in runners with high arches.

Neutral pronation – When the foot lands on the outer edge, then rolls inwards with the ankle remaining straight above the heel and distributing the impact evenly.

Once you know your gait, you'll be able to get advice on the best running shoe for you – this means a shoe that will make your running experience more comfortable, more effective and will help you avoid injury. All specialist local running shops will offer gait analysis, as will bigger chains like Runners Need, who have stores around the UK. It is usually free as part of the fitting service when you're buying running shoes but is also sometimes offered for a small fee (around £15) as a standalone service.

Getting the right shoe is so important that some running shops/brands even offer a forty-five- or ninety-day free trial in which you can return trainers if you're not happy with them and get a full refund.

WARNING: PUBLIC TREADMILL RUNNING

If you've never had your gait analysis done, I feel like I should prepare you. You see, in order for your gait to be analysed, they have to record your feet while you run on a treadmill. I was *mortified* the first time I did this. There I was, in the middle of a busy shop, surrounded by normal shoppers going about their normal business, when the sales assistant turned to me.

'If you could just step onto the treadmill and run at a normal pace,' he said.

'OK,' I said. Then a voice in my head screamed, *Argh!*

Not only was the shop full, but the sales assistant's computer was right at my backside and he was sat there, just watching. I felt the redness creeping up my neck as I started to run.

I'm so embarrassed, I thought.

Then I started thinking about my feet. They were being watched. Suddenly I felt super conscious. Was I running properly? Was I running right? Should I try to run better?

It was the longest minute of my life.

When I climbed off, I looked around to see if any shoppers were pointing or staring. They weren't, they were too busy looking for new trainers. Then I looked at the sales assistant: did I run wrong and was he laughing at me? Again, no.

'Let me show you how your foot moves when you run,' he said.

It was *fascinating*. He showed me the way my foot moved from a number of different angles. Turns out my right foot does a funny flick. As it's about to land on the ground, it does a little twisty kick and then it lands straight. I've literally no idea why my right foot is possessed and does a little dance, but it does. Immediately, this gave me a possible reason for some of the injuries and niggles I'd experienced and it helped the sales assistant recommend the shoes that would give me the support I needed. Let me tell you, the difference when I went out for my first run in trainers that had been selected based on my gait analysis was a revelation. If you've picked up running and you're doing more than a couple of runs a month, you really do have to get the right shoes, mainly because if you love running and you get injured and you can't run, it's so excruciatingly frustrating and soul-destroying. You should do everything within your power not to get injured and gait analysis and expert advice is something that you can and should do.

Next time you need new trainers, don't just go for the ones that you think are the pretty colour or coolest style. Get your gait analysis, find the ones that fit you and that support you where you need it. Then get *those* in the pretty colour or coolest style.

GAIT ANALYSIS DOS AND DON'TS

To the uninitiated, getting your gait analysis done in the middle of a store with people shopping around you can feel really weird, and you don't really know what to do with yourself. Here's a few hints to make that first time a little bit less awkward …

* DON'T be embarrassed. Despite how it feels, no one is looking at your backside or laughing at the way you run. If anything, they'll look over and think, *oh, they're getting their feet done, what a good idea. I'm going to do that*. Once you've done it once (and had the benefit of finding the perfect trainers), you'll never look back.

* DO tell the sales assistant about anything you're training for or any injuries/issues you might have had in the past as it helps them to build a full picture so they can make the best recommendation.

* DON'T try and run 'better' or 'right' on the treadmill. If you don't run the way you *actually* run, you won't get the right shoe and you will end up with injuries. We are all unique and all run a bit weird – gait analysis helps us find a shoe that supports our individual running style.

* DO try to get your gait analysis done once a year. The more you run, the more your movement will naturally change.

* DO get a running shoe that is half a size to a size larger than your normal shoes. Your feet move and swell as you run, so they need the wiggle room!

* DON'T base the comfort/fit of a pair of trainers just on how they feel walking around on the shop floor, take them for a spin on the treadmill before you buy.

SUPPLEMENTS

These can really help your running and they don't have to be massively complicated. There are a few supplements that I swear by for general health and recovery and some that I find most useful for long runs and races.

Energy gels and chews

Once you start running for longer periods of time energy gels and chews are a great addition to your running kit. A bit of science here: your body uses fat and carbohydrates as fuel sources to feed your muscles when you run. Fat is readily available, *but* it takes longer for the body to break down. This is why carbohydrates are your body's primary fuel source and why they're so important to us runners.

Carbohydrates are stored as glycogen in the muscles, but we can only store a certain amount, which means your glycogen stores deplete as you run. This is where gels and chews come in – they're a fast and easy way to replenish your carbohydrates while out on longer runs. Now, I personally only tend to use these while training for a big run like a marathon, but some people swear by them on all longer runs. As a general rule, you might need gels for high-intensity runs (like hill repeats or intervals) lasting more than sixty minutes or low/moderate-intensity runs at a normal pace that last longer than ninety minutes.

Some gels/chews also include some caffeine for an extra kick and there's lots of different flavours. Just make sure you don't start using gels on a Race Day, train with them to see how they affect your gut and see what suits you best. You don't want to try a gel on Race Day and end up with a stomach ache that will hinder you.

It's worth mentioning that gels aren't essential, but they are convenient. You can get your carbs through other snacks. Cyclists do the same with flapjacks, but let me tell you, it's quite hard to run and chew a slab of flapjack (and you probably won't want to stop to eat as it will affect your time …).

Electrolyte drinks, sachets and chews

When we run, we sweat. And when we sweat, we lose our main electrolyte, sodium. You'll realise this most when you lick your lips after a long run and feel and taste the salty crust.

Electrolytes are vital because they hydrate the body, regulate our nerve and muscle function, and help rebuild damaged tissue (among other functions). And get this, we can also deplete our natural sodium levels if we drink too much water too. This is why replacing electrolytes is so important for runners.

You can take electrolytes in drink or powder/salt form, the latter being added to water before drinking, or as chews. They help to hydrate the body optimally when running, prevent cramps and make sure we have the level of electrolytes we need.

Protein powder

As you probably know, a healthy, balanced diet should contain carbohydrates, fats and protein, the latter being super important for runners. Protein is made up of amino acids, which are used to build and repair muscles and bones, as well as produce hormones and enzymes. A lot of us don't get enough protein from food sources like chicken, fish and pulses so that's where protein powder comes in.

There are lots of fantastic flavours and there's even a much wider range of products derived from plant-based sources for vegetarians, vegans and those who are lactose intolerant. When you pick a protein powder, look for high-quality ingredients and a product that is mainly protein – you don't want products that are full of fillers, additives and sweeteners. Remember, protein powder is a supplement. You should get most of your protein from real food sources and the powder should be used to get that little bit extra.

Multivitamins

If you're eating a healthy, balanced diet then you will get most of your vitamins and minerals from the food you eat. Multivitamins are just a good way to fill any gaps or short-falls. Pick a multivitamin that contains well-known nutrients like vitamin C, calcium, iron and potassium, as well as thiamine, riboflavin and niacin, vitamins B6, B12 and folate, magnesium, selenium and zinc, vitamins A, E and K, and vitamin D2 or D3.

Collagen

Breakthrough research in recent years has identified the benefits of collagen not just for recovery and muscle growth after exercise but also it can help promote good joint and bone health, and support lean muscle mass. I started taking collagen to support my running back in 2009 while training for my first marathon. Collagen is a protein that supports the health of your skin, muscles, bones, tendons, ligaments and other connective tissues – all the stuff we rely on to run. So, if your body doesn't have enough, you'll find it harder to recover and may be more prone to injury. Once I started taking it, I was so impressed with the benefits. I wanted to take a higher dose to see better results and in the end co-founded my own health brand, Kollo Health. Our first product was Kollo Collagen, a premium liquid marine collagen supplement that I created with runners in mind (although to be fair it's a great whole-body supplement for absolutely everyone) ...

HYDRATION VEST

If there's one piece of kit that I wish I'd started using sooner, it's a hydration vest. These are basically just very compact backpacks designed to fit like a vest that you can carry your water – usually between 5–15 litres – and other stuff with you on a run. Whenever I'd see a runner wearing one, I'd just think, *oh, they must be proper serious*, because they look so slick and professional. I was so sure they weren't for runners like me that I didn't actually get one until 2022 – can you believe it?

Let me tell you, they are a game changer and you don't need to be a pro to feel the benefits. I hate carrying things when I run and a hydration vest resolves that. There are lots of different types across a broad price range, suitable for short runs and for much longer ones, and some also have extra space to carry other bits you need, like your keys, phone, lip balm and money.

Take some time to do the research to find out what suits your specific needs. For example, I find that the flavour of some of my electrolyte sachets can be a bit much if that's all I have to drink so I have a hydration vest that has two chambers for liquid and I put my electrolyte drink in one and just plain water in the other – problem solved! You can get one that you can either store water bottles in pouches in the front, which then connect to tubes you drink through, or a refillable water 'bladder' that you slide into the back of your vest and drink through a long rubber tube – instant refreshment and no swishy water sounds from a bottle in your hand, causing the need to pee!

RUNNING BELTS AND PHONE HOLDERS

These are great for when you're ready to stop stuffing your belongings into your bra, pants and any available pockets. They come in all shapes and sizes and are perfect for carrying your essentials, like gels, keys and lip balm. Running belts sit comfortably on the waist while most phone holders sit on the upper arm. Some use reflective material for running in darker conditions too, so they can be multipurpose – it's just about finding what's best for you.

ICE BATHS AND MASSAGE GUNS

When you start running more and taking on longer distances, recovery becomes even more important. While nothing can compare to booking a regular sports massage to loosen you up, you can deal with niggles and boost recovery by using a handheld massage gun on sore muscles and this is something you can do easily at home. (But be warned: if you have kids, it may be used as a weapon of tickle and torment if left lying around – or at least it is in our house!)

Another option for home recovery is an ice bath. Now you don't need to install a full-on permanent fixture with all the whistles and bells. There are other (simpler) options. You could simply run a bath with cold water, add some ice and there you go.

An alternative is to get an actual ice bath. They're becoming quite the garden accessory just like a shed, bbq or outdoor dining table. However, they really can help reduce muscle soreness after exercise, and many runners swear by them. I know, I am one of them! Ice baths come in all shapes, sizes, materials and prices. For instance, you could invest in a super fancy metal bath which is so cold you have to break the ice to enter the water. Then again, perhaps you'd rather opt for a wooden tub which comes with a temperature control system so you can set it to what works for you (I go between 10 and 15 degrees). You could even get one that fits two people so you and your other half can hold hands while chilling ... how romantic!

Alternatively, you could pick up an inflatable bath. They're not quite as robust but they can still work brilliantly and will save you a chunk of money. It's like a paddling pool for runners. I like to use my ice bath post run and I aim to stay in for between five and fifteen minutes, depending on how I feel, how much time I have and how cold it is! I can testify though that the hardest part is getting in the water, after that it does get easier. A word of warning: ice baths aren't suitable for everyone, so if you're unsure, check with your GP before taking a dip.

ADVANCED KIT LIST

Now that your running has progressed, you can build on the basic kit list I shared on page 17, adding the items below as they become relevant to you:

* Trainers based on gait analysis
* Activity-specific footwear (e.g. trail running shoes)
* Branded or specialist running wear
* Running belt
* Phone holder
* Hydration vest
* Supplements: Energy gels/chews, electrolytes, multi-vitamins, protein powders, collagen supplements
* Ice bath
* Handheld massager.

Now, if you really want to get serious about your kit, there's an annual show that I highly recommend you visit. It's the National Running Show, whose main event takes place in January at the Birmingham NEC – perfect for if you're planning a spring race.

Founded by *RunPod* guest Mike Seaman, it really is like a sweet shop for runners of any level, with lots of stands, from clothing and tech to nutrition and supplements (you might even see me over at the Kollo Health stand). There are inspirational speakers, tons of information on the latest cutting-edge technologies and of course loads and loads of lovely new trainers to look at!

COMPLEMENT YOUR TRAINING

As well as upgrading your kit, there are things that you can do outside of your regular runs that will help you build up speed, endurance, distances, fitness levels and might even help to reduce your risk of injury.

Tracking your stats

Speaking of run times, you only have to watch the start of any mass event – from the London Marathon to a local Saturday parkrun (see also page 198) – to know how much runners love analysing their run data. As you cross the start line, the head goes down, the arms come up and

BEEP, you·start tracking! It's part of the ritual.

If you're ramping up from novice level, you'll almost certainly be more interested in the timing of your runs, among other stats, which means you might want to invest in a running or fitness watch. Before deciding what watch or tracker you get, it's important to understand the main statistics that we runners love to obsess over and analyse:

Distance – Nice and simple, just how far you've travelled on your run. Early on, you'll probably measure this in metres and kilometres, but before you know it, you'll be racking up whole miles!

Time – Another simple one: how long you have run for. Both time and distance are the basic metrics that inform the stats that tell us more about our performance.

Pace – Simply the speed that you run when running, it's usually stated as minutes per mile or minutes per kilometre.

Average Pace – The average speed you were running at over the entire distance of your run, regardless of if you varied your speed at points throughout the run. It can be calculated by dividing your run time (in minutes and seconds) by the distance of your run (kilometres or miles).

Split Pace – A running and racing term that refers to the time that it takes to complete a key distance. So, if it takes you six minutes to run 1km, then your split pace is six minutes per kilometre. You might break a 5K down into 1K splits or a marathon into 5K splits. Splits allow you to see if you're running at a consistent speed, pacing yourself over your run. Positive splits are when you run each 'split' more slowly than the last. Negative splits, which is what lots of runners aim for, mean that you run each split faster than the last.

Elevation – This is how high you climbed during a run. You'll be surprised how many sneaky hills there are on even a route that seems quite flat!

Cadence – The number of steps you take per minute while running. It's also sometimes called step or stride frequency.

Heart Rate – This is the number of times your heart beats per minute and is an indicator of the intensity of your run. Average heart rates vary from person to person due to factors such as age, weight and general fitness levels, but a normal resting heart rate is usually sixty to a hundred beats per minute. When running, it's usually between a hundred and 160.

Heart Rate Variability (HRV) – When your heart beats, there's usually a different amount of time between beats and some are faster/slower than others. HRV is the measurement of this variation in time between heartbeats and it's a good indicator of how your body is functioning and recovering. By analysing your HRV, you can see if you need more rest or are ready to go. Some fitness trackers use HRV to inform a 'readiness' or 'body battery' score.

VO2 Max – There's a lot that you can delve into with this, which I'm not going to go into here. But to explain it simply, VO2 Max is a measure of your aerobic fitness – the maximum amount of oxygen your body can absorb and use during exercise. An increase in VO2 = an improvement in your cardiovascular capacity. This is a detailed measurement that some runners love to track and analyse, but I'm not one of them!

CHOOSING A RUNNING WATCH/ FITNESS TRACKER

Looking at all the available options can be overwhelming and the cost can vary wildly. As with picking the right trainers, it's a personal thing and the most expensive doesn't necessarily = the best for you. There are some stats and metrics that you might not care about. For me, I'm not bothered or interested to know about my cadence. Some people love geeking out on it, but it's just not for me. All I'm really interested in (aside from the obvious distance and time) is pace and heart rate. It took me a while to understand pace but now it's what stops me from running too slow or – more importantly – too fast, so I don't burn out. I would also love a watch that had a speedometer, like a treadmill does, so I can see exactly how fast I'm going, rather than working out pace, but I'm still waiting for a tracker that has that dream feature!

When choosing a running watch/fitness tracker, consider the following things:

* What are the stats that matter to you? – If you just want to get a general overview of your daily activity and general fitness, a basic fitness watch will probably be suitable as this will tell you your step count, calories and distance. If you want more detail on your distance, pace and time then a mid-range watch will be better for you.

* Do you want heart rate data? – Make sure the watch or tracker you choose has a heart rate monitor (HRM).

* Do you want GPS? – If accuracy is important, GPS watch data tends to be more accurate. It also allows you to map your runs.

* Do you want to track advanced stats? – If you really want to get into the nitty-gritty of your running data and look

at things like VO2 Max, then you'll need a mid-range or advanced model.

※ Do you do other sports that you may wish to track data for? – A multisport watch might be more suitable than a dedicated running watch. If you also swim, water resistance is important too.

※ Will you wear it just to run, or all the time? – Sounds daft, but if it's going to be your main watch, it needs to look nice!

※ What apps do you want to use with it? – If you use apps to track your runs, you might want to check that you can connect those apps to your smartwatch.

STRENGTH EXERCISES

When you LOVE running, sometimes it's the only thing that you want to do. But when you run frequently, it's really important to strengthen your body through other exercises too, which is where strength and conditioning training comes in.

Strength and conditioning training involves a series of dynamic (involving movement) and static (holding the same position) exercises, which can be done with weights or without – using just your bodyweight instead. They help to improve movement and mobility and physical performance, as well as your general health. For runners, strength training will:

* Help you use oxygen more efficiently, improving your performance

* Help you to run faster by boosting co-ordination and power

* Help prevent injuries by strengthening muscles and connective tissues.

Another thing to think about is that when you run, you are only training one part of your body. Your quads, hamstrings and calves do most of the work, along with your hips and glutes; upper body – shoulders and arms – may help, but they're not getting a full workout.

Lifting weights not only allows you to strengthen your core and upper body, improve posture and balance, avoiding muscle imbalance and potential injury, it will allow you to even out any imbalances in your lower body too – we all have a stronger leg and single-leg (or unilateral) exercises can help us address those.

There are several ways to bring strength training into your routine. If you are training for a particular goal or race, it might be worth enlisting the support of a strength and conditioning coach to tailor your training plan specifically to your needs and keep you accountable. However, this can be expensive in the long term so other options to consider are:

* Book a session with a personal trainer (PT) at your local gym and ask them to create a strength and conditioning plan that you can follow. Some gyms even offer a free one-off session to get you started.

* Check out online fitness sessions and programmes on YouTube, Sky and other on-demand TV services. They have lots of at-home and bodyweight workouts you can try.

* Do a home-based session using the exercises I recommend below. You can do this using your bodyweight, but if you want to make it harder, buy some free weights and bands to use at home. Remember to start light and work up as your strength improves, go too heavy, too fast and you'll risk injury. If you want to save money, you could chip in with friends and share the weights.

STRENGTH EXERCISES

Now, these exercises certainly aren't my favourites, but they're the ones I find to be most beneficial – why not give them a go a couple of times a week on your non-running days?

Before you start, if you do have any specific health conditions or injuries you should talk to your GP or an advanced or clinical exercise instructor, as some of these exercises might not be suitable.

Jump Squats

Truly exhausting, but hugely beneficial for building strength and endurance in the legs – and they're the part of the body doing the running! Try doing twenty Jump Squats, aiming to go as low as possible, and then rest for two minutes. Repeat three times.

Single-Leg Squats

It sounds simple enough, but I know you'll hate me for this one! Try getting up from a stool, chair or a bench on one leg, then sit back down and repeat. Do twelve reps on each leg, then rest for two minutes before going again. Repeat three times.

Walking Lunges

A dynamic version of a static lunge. Instead of standing back upright after doing a lunge on one leg, you move forward by performing a lunge with the other leg instead. Walking across a room or outdoor space, do twenty lunges forward and back. Rest for two minutes then repeat three times. To make this harder, add weight by carrying a dumbbell in each hand.

Lunge Jumps

Lunge jumps are a plyometric exercise, which is essentially anything involving short, intense bursts of activity that target fast-twitch muscle fibres in the lower body. These fibres help generate explosive power that increases speed and jumping height. Plyometric exercises are amazing for us all and will really complement your running. Lunge jumps are a progression of a standard lunge, where you jump high in the air and switch your forward foot before landing. Do ten on each leg and alternate as you go, so this would mean twenty in total. Rest for two minutes. Repeat three times.

Glute Bridges

Glute work is important, so try Glute Bridges. Lie on your back and lift your hips upwards, hold your glutes tight, then slowly lower back down again. This not only strengthens your glutes, but also increases core stability and lower back health too. Repeat the movement twelve to fifteen times, then rest for two minutes. Repeat three times.

To progress the exercise, place a weight on your hips or make it even harder by lifting one leg up in the air, so it's a Single-Leg Glute Bridge … OUCH!

Step-Ups

Get a bench or chair and step up and down in a steady and controlled manner. When stepping, don't let the other leg take any weight, it should all be on the stepping leg. Do this ten times on each leg, then rest for two minutes. Repeat three times.

This exercise can be progressed and made harder by

holding a dumbbell in each hand, increasing the weight as your strength improves.

Side Plank

A great exercise for the hips, legs and core, simply hold your body on your side in a straight position supported only by one arm and the side of one foot. If this is a bit too hard, you can keep the side of your knee on the floor and raise the hip only. Hold the position for thirty to forty seconds each side. Rest. Repeat three times.

Clamshells

Lie on one side, with your ankles together, propped up on one arm. Hinging at the hip and ankle, lift your top knee up and then lower it back down to the bottom knee. You can add resistance by putting a band above your knees, which is great for glute activation and to target hip abductor muscles. Do twenty reps each side then rest. Repeat three times.

Press-Ups

Running is all about the legs, but don't neglect the upper body. Press-ups are great for upper body arm and chest strength. If you can't do a press-up on your hands and toes, you can start on your knees, leaning on a bench and then progress from there. Aim for ten to fifteen press-ups (or as many as you can get). Rest for two minutes. Repeat three times.

If you're struggling to achieve even a few press-ups on your knees, try Shoulder Taps instead. Get into a high-plank position, with your legs extended straight back and your shoulders, elbows and wrists all in a straight line. Engage your core then lift your right hand off the floor and touch your left shoulder. Repeat with the left hand. Make sure you keep your hips still and stable as you repeat ten times on each side (twenty taps in total). Rest for two minutes. Repeat three times.

The thing to remember about strength training is that as well as for running, strength training is brilliant for you, regardless of age, gender or whether you're a runner or not. It's a simple fact that if you're not strength training now, you probably won't be able to get off the loo seat without a struggle when you're older, so I'd recommend it to everyone!

YOGA

When I was training for the London Marathon before I had Ella, I was also doing two ninety-minute Ashtanga Yoga sessions a week on my non-running days.

I found that cross-training with yoga stopped everything from being tight for my next run, making it a bit easier and more enjoyable. Yoga can also help build muscle, strengthen your lower and upper body and core, and promotes relaxation, so it's pretty great all round. It really did supplement my training when I was at my very fittest, running four days a week and training in the gym twice a week. But back then, I didn't have a child, I wasn't working six days a week and I had more time on my hands! If it's something you enjoy and you can fit it in, I would certainly recommend yoga, but you can definitely build and improve on your fitness without it.

SET GOALS AND GET A TRAINING PLAN

Starting out, your running goals tend to focus very much on just getting out there and getting your run done, consistently. But once you're doing that, your goals shift up a gear. You may decide you want to build up distance, or that you're going to do a race for the first time.

Building up distance

You might have mastered your 5K route and feel ready to push yourself further but just because 10K is the next distance up, don't go out and try and get it on your first go. If you do that, you'll risk injuring yourself *and* denting your confidence. The trick is to build it up, step by step:

* Allow yourself eight to twelve weeks to make the transition.

* Only increase your total distance by 10 per cent each week.

* Cross-train and give your legs a rest. Integrate another form of exercise that you enjoy in order to build on your general fitness – swimming, strength training and yoga or Pilates all work well.

* Do interval training for one run per week to start improving your endurance.

* Complete one longer run per week.

* Take rest days, so your muscles can recover.

* Set yourself a goal to keep you focused – maybe even sign up for a race.

Taking on a race

If you've never done a race before, a 5 or 10K is the perfect place to start and a great motivator for your training. Planning for a race involves the same principles of goal setting that I discussed earlier in Chapter 2 (see also page 37) – working backwards from the intended outcome and planning the steps you need to take in-between. However, when planning for a race, rather than just scheduling runs, you're actually creating a training plan.

In training plans for running races of any distance you will build up to your longest run before you start to 'taper' towards the end of the plan with some shorter runs. Tapering is important because it allows you to build up endurance, then gives your mind and body time to recover from that hard training. That way you'll be ready and rested for the race and have more energy to draw on.

Training plans are incredibly personal and individual as they take in factors like your age, running experience, previous injuries and your lifestyle and routine. If you want something highly personalised, you could try a running coach. Often there are personal trainers in gyms who specialise in running, you might even find one locally through an online search – or the best are often word of mouth. There are varying degrees of coaching – they could essentially hold your hand from day one to your goal, checking in weekly and customising a programme specifically for an event, or they could just write out a training plan for you to work towards.

I have worked a couple of times with a trainer, and it was really useful as they can adapt the running programme as you go, and I have also used running apps – although these are more generalised and less tailored to me and my weekly availability. It really depends what you are willing to invest and how motivated you are without someone telling you what to do. My marathon PB was when I was working with a personal trainer who also designed my running programme. But, if you're just looking for a starting point, you could try my general 10K training plan on page 262, search online and study training plans that are available from reputable running publications like *Runner's World*, sports brands and even health organisations. Or use an app like Runna or Coopah, which allows you to build a training plan in minutes, based on information you provide, such as age, target distance, date of race and how many times a week you run.

COLSON'S STORY

Like so many people, Colson Smith (aka Craig from ITV's *Coronation Street*) found running in 2020 during the first UK lockdown. He started with the singular aim of losing weight, but by his own admission, 'It didn't take very long for the running to become more important than the losing weight bit.' From a first run, as incognito as possible while it was pitch-black one morning to starting trail running and putting races like the Loch Ness and Big Five marathons on his to-do list, Colson came onto *RunPod* in June 2021 to talk about how he ramped up his running.

Speaking of his change of mindset from being weight-loss focused Colson said: 'People can get held up on numbers and hitting numeric goals of weight loss, whereas for me, now, it's completely about the pace that I run at, the time that I can run for. Setting goals like that to become healthier and fitter makes you happier.'

He went on, 'Setting those small goals of "I want to run this quickly" or "I want to lift this much weight" makes everything so much easier because when you hit those goals, you just get on to setting the next ones and it's constantly about just achieving things for yourself.'

When I asked Colson when he realised that running was more than just a way to lose weight, he mentioned that his ever-increasing collection of running shoes gave the game away. But what exactly was it that made him realise that he was a runner?

'You start buying all the gear, don't you? So, you start off in a scratty pair of trainers and then you're there with trail shoes – quick shoes – and it all kind of comes together,' he explained. 'But I think, for me, it will have taken me a good four or five months to say, "Do you know what? I deserve to run now" and it's a weird thing that clicks. I guess I was running purely to lose weight and then when I realised that I liked running and I was running to become a better runner. I think that's when I went, "Oh, I am a runner now".

'I never thought I'd have a running watch. I absolutely love my Garmin, wear it every day, and I listen to it. It helps me with my training, helps me with everything. But I have got a vest, which is called a "naked" vest, and it basically is for trails, so I put my gels and stuff in the back, I put my water in the front,' he continued. 'I never thought I would be a guy to invest in a vest to run in. It's almost like a thermal compression top that you put on over what you're wearing and you put your bottles in the front and everything else in your back, but you don't feel like you've got anything on.'

As well as sharing advice on kit, Colson also gave some brilliant advice for newer runners wishing to improve their running.

'When you've got past the bit of doing it for yourself and when you're enjoying running, when you decide you want to go out to run regularly, getting a bit of a plan and some purpose behind your run is definitely worth doing,' he said. 'Now I do between three and four runs a week. I make sure I do one base run, which is really easy, at a pace that I could run at all day and just enjoy myself. Then I do one tempo run, where I try to run a bit quicker and then I do a long run.

'One thing that I have added in, which I absolutely love, is trail running. It's just something that was completely different. You don't worry about pace, you don't look at your watch all the time, you don't listen to music, you just go, and you chat. You're running up hills and you're walking a bit and you're talking and you're taking it easy, and you don't realise how much work you're doing. For me, I found that it massively improved my fitness.

'Then every now and then, I'll chuck in a really quick 5K and I use that as a way to monitor how far my progression is coming on, but now in the really geeky way, all my gym sessions I do to become a better runner. I decided that I wanted to make sure I've got stronger legs and stronger ankles so that I can run more and that I can run faster – I have gone full geek, haven't I?'

You have, Colson. It comes to us all – and it's brilliant. Here's to achieving goals and loving the journey!

6

SLOWING DOWN TO SPEED UP

When you really get into running, it's tempting to spend all your time hammering away and working hard, trying to shave seconds off a personal best (PB) or just trying to make every run faster than the last. You might see your friends or other runners doing races, winning medals and getting better times, and feel the pressure to sprint out of the door for every single run so you can 'keep up with the Joneses'. But unless you're actively training for a big event yourself, or you're a professional runner, do you *really* need to hit it that hard all the time? Sometimes routine and comparison to others can diminish the joy of running and the fact that going for a run is supposed to be an enjoyable thing can easily be forgotten.

Now, in my experience, pushing yourself on every

single run will not only exhaust you, but it can cause you to lose the love for running and even be detrimental to your performance too. That's why slowing down is sometimes the smart choice.

WHAT IS A SLOW RUN?

As always with running, this is very individual. A slow run for you might be a sprint for someone else, but there are a couple of guidelines for what a slow run is.

If you know your pace, a slow run is generally considered to be one to three minutes per mile slower than your 10K pace, or at least one to two minutes per mile slower than marathon pace. If you're not sure of your pace or don't measure it, another way to work out if you're actually running slowly is to see if you can talk while running. By the way, I'm not talking about a few gasped sentences here – if you are truly running slowly, you should be able to hold a full conversation comfortably as you go!

NO SHAME IN A SLOW JOG

Sometimes I do decide to do a slow, gentle run and I love running so much when I do this. I get a chance to look around, chill out and concentrate on my breathing and it reignites my passion for running. You should try and do it every now and then.

There's nothing wrong in wanting to get better at running, but improvements and achievements don't always have to be hard-won times or tough distances. You can also take the time to appreciate what you now consider to be an 'easy' run – could you do that 'easy' thirty-minute run quite so effortlessly a few months ago, or would you have struggled?

This kind of achievement is just as amazing as hitting a PB, believe me!

You should also consider what your goals are. Sure, if you're training for a 5K, 10K or even a marathon and you want to hit a specific time, maybe you're going to need to do some harder runs. But what if you just want to complete a distance. Is there as much need to push yourself?

As running becomes an increasingly broad church, with people of all levels of fitness and all types of goals getting involved, running times are actually getting slower. The average finish time for a parkrun 5K in 2005 was twenty-two minutes seventeen seconds. In 2023, it was thirty-two minutes thirty-four seconds. There's a greater acceptance that as well as people who may need to run slowly, due to injury or health reasons, there are those who *want* to run slowly too.

In 2020, in consultation with slower runners, the London Marathon launched a new 'back-of-the-pack' initiative which saw the finish line on The Mall remain open until 7.30 p.m. and the introduction of tailwalkers going at eight-hour marathon pace walking at the back of the final wave, with drink stations and timing mats remaining in place until the tailwalkers passed, so even slower runners got the full marathon experience[10].

You definitely don't have to run fast to enjoy it. Sometimes all you need is a bit of exercise, which is good for your head and good for your heart. That gets the colour in your cheeks and makes you sweat a bit.

We don't always have to be pushing ourselves to achieve something. We don't have to be training intensely. Sometimes we can just go at a pace we enjoy and it's great that even events/races like parkrun and the London Marathon are now accommodating this kind of running too. There really is no shame in a slow jog!

LISTEN TO YOUR BODY

One weekend last summer, I spent seven hours in the continuous rain, at a golf tournament, followed by another eight hours the following day in rain, thunder and lightning and strong winds, with minimal sleep and a two-hour drive either side. The next day I was at work first thing as normal and planning to do my usual run commute. But as I got started, I noticed how every movement was heavy and cumbersome. I wasn't out of breath, but my legs were dragging. It was like wading through treacle. Rather than feeling re-invigorated like I usually do, I was yawning and just feeling more and more tired. My body was telling me that it was not the day for a run so instead of pushing for my usual pace, I stopped and walked the rest of the way home. It wasn't my best, but it was the best I could manage in the situation.

Listening to what your body is telling you is important if you want to keep the love of running and avoid injuries. I'm all for a bit of 'no pain no gain' attitude, but sometimes pain is a sign that something's not right and that you need to rest. Sometimes, though, it's not your body having its say. It's your mind – and that's where things can get tricky.

On occasion after leaving for work at 5 a.m., doing my radio show and finishing at 10 a.m., I'll sometimes find myself about to start my run and think, *No, I'm just too knackered*. But before I throw in the towel, I really have to question what I'm feeling.

Is it just because I've been up early and not had much sleep? I know I can run my way through that and I'll feel better in the end. Is it because I'm genuinely broken or I really just can't be bothered?

Do I genuinely not want to run, or am I making an excuse?

You might recognise that feeling. Or maybe, also like me, you'll remember a time you looked at a big rain cloud in the sky, or clock showing you're setting off later than expected and asked a friend, colleague or partner (who was not running): 'Do you think I should do this run or not?'

If you're asking this question, I guarantee you will want them to say 'No, leave it' and more often than not, they will. Why? Because they will feel better because that way neither of you are running. No one has bragging rights. Now, if you ask someone who is about to exercise, with you or otherwise, I guarantee they will usually say, 'Yes, just give it a go.' Sometimes *who* you ask to make such a decision is as telling as *what* you're asking.

For those times when I'm not quite sure if my body is telling me I need to take it easy, or my mind is telling me I can't be bothered (despite being perfectly ready and able to run), I have a tactic: I make a deal with myself. I have to set off as normal and at least try. If, after one mile, I'm not feeling it, if my legs are heavy and I've had to walk, then I know it's my body giving me a message. From there I'll either walk home because I think being outside will benefit me, or I'll just get on the tube. But if the fog clears and I get through those difficult first few minutes, I know it was my mind telling me that I didn't feel like running, even though I was perfectly fine to do so. I'll be pleased that I gave it a go and will be running happily along, all the way home, feeling great. You see, your mind plays tricks on you, but your body doesn't. Seeing how I get on in those first few minutes is a little test I have for my body.

RELAX INTENTIONALLY

If you do decide to listen to your body and maybe take a day off from running, or any exercise, whatever you do, DON'T spend the whole day feeling guilty about it. Decide what day you will next run or exercise, commit it to the diary and then forget about it, until the time comes. Once that's out of your head, you can be intentional in how you relax.

Go to bed early, loaf on the sofa, meditate, journal, read, cook, or bake, scroll on your phone, watch TV, play games … whatever it is that gives you peace and relaxation, just do it and let go of any guilt about not running. There's no point in sitting around thinking about what you should have been doing. The fact is if you'd forced yourself to do the run against your body's wishes, you'd probably have hated it, it would have been miserable and you really wouldn't have got anything out of it.

Here's a few things I do when I skip a run and want to be intentional about how I use that time:

Watch a movie – At the cinema or at home on the sofa, curled up with the dog.

Walk the dog – It's a different pace but I'm still outside so still active, just not pushing myself.

Clear out a cupboard – It might sound weird but sometimes to take my mind off being active and force myself to relax, I clear out a cupboard. Honestly, it's crazy how therapeutic it can be.

Face mask or foot mask – To be honest, these happen rarely but they are a good way to force yourself to stop, sit down and relax. You can all too easily forget to look after yourself and as much as tidying the house, making dinner and getting things organised at home are important, when you have some free time, a little self-care is highly recommended. It forces you to relax, switch off (at least a bit) and enjoy doing nothing. What's more, if it's a foot mask you've opted for, your toes might thank you for it too – after all the running I do, my feet desperately need some TLC!

SLOWING DOWN TO RECOVER

Now, many of us are committed to training because we love it and because we have a target, so we're really reluctant to take our foot off the gas. But whether you're training intensely for a particular goal, or just running to get healthier, your body still needs a rest. This is exactly why we have rest days and recovery runs.

Rest days – Days without running (or perhaps any exercise) at all allow your muscles time to rebuild and strengthen.

You replenish your glycogen stores ahead of your next session and avoid injuries like stress fractures that can be caused by over-training.

Some people choose to do other exercises on 'rest days', such as a gentle walk or some strength training, but you really should have at least one day per week without any exercise at all to allow your body and mind to relax and replenish.

Recovery runs – These are slow, easy-paced runs that should follow tougher, more intensive runs in your training plan, like tempo runs and intervals, or after Race Days. These should be very low-intensity runs of no more than twenty to thirty minutes to truly help you to recover.

THE IMPORTANCE OF SLEEP

If we're talking about rest and recovery for running, here we must discuss the importance of sleep. It's not just a case of not feeling too tired to run, sleep is crucial to performance.

* Sleep strengthens the immune system – If you have a good immune system, you're less likely to get sick and be forced not to run. In reducing the risk of illness, you'll also be able to run more consistently, which will help improve running performance.

* Sleep repairs damage and helps build muscles and bones – When you sleep after exercise, growth hormones are released. These help to repair cellular and tissue damage from exercise and prepare the body better for your next session.

* Sleep supports good cardiovascular health – Getting enough sleep can also lower the risk of heart disease and stroke.

* Sleep helps fight fatigue – A good night's sleep means you'll have the energy needed to complete your run and may even go faster if you've rested and recovered well enough.

You only have to look at pro athletes across all disciplines to see this in action. Former world number one tennis player Sir Andy Murray slept twelve hours a day at the height of his game[11]. US champion tennis player Venus Williams sleeps up to ten hours a day[12] and one of the greatest runners in the world, Kenyan long-distance runner Eliud Kipchoge, sleeps for eight hours at night and takes a two-hour nap during the day to get the sleep required for performance[13]. In many cases professional athletes prioritise sleep over a whole host of other things – and with good reason. But most of us don't have the luxury of guaranteeing ourselves twelve undisturbed hours of shuteye a night.

Despite the fact healthy adults are advised to get seven

to nine hours of sleep per night, in order to function at their best, one in five people in the UK (35 per cent) only get six hours or less[14]. So why is it that we think we can still deliver run after run at high intensity on top of our full-time jobs and minimal sleep, while also running around after the kids, doing all the washing, cooking the dinner …? It's craziness.

While we should certainly all strive for those seven to nine hours per night, runners or not, I know it's not always possible. The nature of my own work and lifestyle, with early starts and lots of family and other commitments, has always meant that getting the right amount of sleep is a challenge. Many times, I have had to sacrifice getting the right amount of sleep to enable me to have the time in my day to do the run at all.

Understanding the importance of sleep and how it affects my running means that I know when I decide to run on a less-than-optimal amount of sleep, my performance might not be at its best. I might not go my furthest or be at my fastest, but getting the run done and getting my high from the satisfaction of that is more important to me – it's a pay-off. Understanding why I might not be as fast or find it as easy also helps relieve the frustration around perfor-mance as I know I've made a conscious decision about what's most important to me and it lets me just enjoy the run for what it is.

SLOWING DOWN TO SPEED UP

If there's anything that might convince the more goal-orientated of you of the benefits of slowing down your running, let it be research led by Dr Stephen Seiler, a globally renowned exercise physiologist at the University of Agder in Norway. He found that elite athletes train around 80 per cent of the time at low intensity and just 20 per cent at high intensity[15].

If we're so keen to adopt their favourite trainers, gels and running gear, we should probably be taking a leaf out of elite athletes' training books too, right? The fact of the matter is that incorporating slow runs actually helps us to speed up and become better runners:

* You'll run with less effort on faster, harder run days – Easy runs train the cardiovascular and respiratory systems, and your muscles to work more efficiently and integrate better, which will make even your hard runs seem easier.

* You'll build up your aerobic system – Faster anaerobic runs mainly use stored muscle glycogen from carbohydrates, but slow aerobic runs use approximately 80 per cent fat for energy. This will eventually make longer distance runs more sustainable and you'll need to refuel less as your body uses fat as its main fuel source rather than carbs.

* You can focus on technique – When you're running slowly, you have more time to think about your form.

Improved running form helps you run more efficiently, which over time will help you run further and faster.

⁎ You'll reduce the risk of injury – Slow running helps strengthen your joints, bones, tendons and ligaments. This helps them to adapt to the stress of running without going at a pace that might cause injury.

THE 'SUNDAY RUN'

The slow run also plays an important role in *any* running training plan. Regardless of what distance you are training for, you don't go out there and do three runs a week, of exactly the same distance at exactly the same pace. You'll have a fast, high-intensity run and most likely run intervals for another, both of which will improve your overall fitness levels, and then the third run will almost certainly be long and slow. Often called the 'Sunday Run' as that's the day most people have the time available to do a longer run at a slow pace, it might feel easy but it's actually helping you to improve your running. The Sunday Run is the run that will get you your distance, that will build endurance and really test how far you can go.

By the way, you don't have to do the Sunday Run on a Sunday. You can do it whenever you have time! Mine is usually done on a Monday because Sunday is the day I take off to spend with family and enjoy slobbing on the sofa.

LOW HEART-RATE TRAINING

Another example of slower running that can improve your performance and endurance is low heart-rate training. This style of training was pioneered by running coach Dr Phil Maffetone[16], who created a formula for the heart rate that you should do your training runs at:

180 – [your age] = Heart rate you should maintain while training (bpm)

If you experienced two or more colds a year, indicating a weaker immune system, then you should deduct a further 5 from the total. So, for me at forty-seven years old at the time of writing, this would mean running at 133 bpm. Now, believe me, running with my heart rate at 133 bpm would feel like I'm practically walking and a gentle jog would send my heart rate well above that rate but it's a really effective way to keep me at a slow jog and great for improving aerobic fitness too.

Low heart-rate training allows you to increase your aerobic capacity without the strain, injuries and illness that can come from over-training. It's quite tough to stick to and you really need to build it up over time, but if you do, then you will eventually be able to run faster with less effort.

This used to be an approach that mainly elite athletes took because the tech wasn't as widely available. But now, as many fitness trackers and running watches have heart-rate monitors and there are also plenty of other pieces of affordable and accessible tech to monitor heart rate, it's open to pretty much anyone to try.

RUNNING FATIGUE

Stopping or slowing down might seem counterintuitive if you have a goal in mind, but sometimes we can be pushing for improvement that isn't really happening and that's when running fatigue may set in. Of course, we all occasionally feel a little tired and achy after a run when we're training. But running fatigue is more severe and can be a sign of over-training. It can feel like being constantly over-tired from training, having muscle pain that makes running difficult, or fighting off lots of injuries and niggles all the time. You'll likely hit a plateau in performance as well.

I went through this myself a few years ago. Every day, I would come out of work and run home the same route, five times a week. I was pushing hard, I was sticking to it, but I wasn't improving. In fact, I actually started to slow down. But it wasn't just that, I was bored. I wasn't enjoying it: I had running fatigue. It was horrible because I was desperate to be doing good, enjoyable runs again, but it just wasn't happening, so I did what for me was unimaginable at the time – I took a little break.

There was a short period of sitting on the sofa, watching TV, scrolling, thinking about running a lot and some feeling guilty. Then I decided to try something different for a little while. Instead of running my same usual route every day, I started going to a workout class again, which combined treadmill running and weights exercises in a circuit. It was great because it was 50 per cent running, 50 per cent weights, but you'd never know how they would split that up – the variety kept me interested.

After a while, I started running home from work again – not every day, but some days. Instead of going hard back on my usual route, I went more steadily on a longer route some days; other days I did hill sprints or intervals. I mixed it up, the boredom started to lift and the enjoyment returned.

Before you get to the point that I did though, there are some ways you can prevent running fatigue:

* Incorporate rest days and recovery runs – Give your muscles time to heal and help to build up your strength and stamina.

* Gradually increase pace or distance – You don't have to go hard all the time and don't have to make big leaps in distance. Only increase your weekly running distance by a maximum of 10 per cent.

* Get enough sleep – Bounce back from the physical and mental impact of your run.

* Eat enough – Make sure you're following a balanced diet and getting enough calories to sustain your activity.

* Stay hydrated – The more dehydrated you are on a run, the more tired you'll be after it. Hydration shouldn't only come just before and during a run, but consistently throughout the day.

* Vary your activities – To prevent mental fatigue and boredom, don't do the same run over and over. Create a training plan with variety, incorporating high- and medium-intensity runs, like hill sprints, Fartleks and intervals, with low-intensity longer runs, recovery runs and other exercise that complements your running, such as yoga, Pilates or strength training (see pages 44-5).

KAREN'S STORY

Runner, triathlete, personal trainer, endurance coach and serial *RunPod* guest Karen Weir loves an easy run. She advocates taking the pressure off so it's easier to get out there and just really enjoy it, without worrying about our performance.

'Obviously, running is a great form of exercise, but if you don't feel like running, walking is as good as,' she said. 'Basically, running is faster walking, or walking is slower running.

'There are many people now, and many coaches, who are pushing the idea of run-walking. If something feels really hard to you, you're less likely to go out the door and do it. But if you give yourself permission that you are going to start with a walk or take walking breaks, the whole exercise feels like it's going to be a little bit easier, then you are going to have that motivation to get out the door.

'If you're just thinking, *I need to go out and run five miles hard*, that takes extra, extra motivation to get out there and do that. But if you say, "I'm going to go out there and do five miles and I'm going to walk every half mile for a minute" or "I'm going to walk for ten minutes to start and gradually build into it", that's so much easier to manage and you get back and you feel just as good.'

So many of us beat ourselves up about not having sufficient willpower or motivation to get out on our run, but Karen thinks that we need more than motivation to keep running in our lives long-term.

'Motivation isn't the answer. Motivation isn't enough. We have to bring in other elements and part of that is having a compelling reason to do what you're doing; to be enjoying what you do, but also you do have to instil discipline and not rely on motivation and willpower because that is not enough. Just knowing that it's not [enough] is a good start, so don't beat yourself up,' she said.

'When we talk about motivation from a psychological perspective there is the idea of extrinsically motivated and intrinsically motivated. If our motivation comes from inside, from the love of doing something, for the joy of trying to improve, we're much more likely to keep something up,' she added. 'Versus if we are extrinsically motivated, which means being motivated by external things, so things like social media and getting kudos and being able to post on Strava and all that, getting a medal, those are external motivations. They might motivate you in a very short term and for a short period of time, but ultimately the intrinsic – the love, the joy of it – is not there and people wonder why they can't carry on.

'To make running part of your life, and a life-long process, you have to make sure you do it in a way that is joyful, that you love doing. That doesn't mean to say that every single run you go out and say, "Yeah, it's brilliant, I'm loving it," but that's where the discipline comes in. You have to say, 80 per cent of the time "I love what I'm doing" and if you don't, stop. Try something else, because there are plenty of other things you can do to stay fit and healthy, and just taking a break can make a difference as well. If you have had an intensive period of training for a marathon or something, there's nothing wrong with taking a couple of months off, doing something else, trying something else.'

So where exactly does Karen find her own runner's high?

'On a nice sunny day when I set myself the goal of just doing an easy, easy run and I just stick to that. I'm not pushing on. I'm taking it easy and not having to work really hard on a run,' she said. 'It's just nice to get to the stage where you think, *OK, it's not hard, but I am still running*, this idea that we have to run hard every time, I'm just not interested in that anymore. I'm interested in easy running – when it *does* feel easy. When you've made it feel easy because you've gone out with that intention to run slowly.'

7

RUNNER'S LOWS AND HOW TO OVERCOME THEM

No matter how much you love running, what you achieve in the sport and how good you get at it, there is no avoiding the fact that it has its lows as well as those amazing highs that we all love so much. These range from minor inconveniences, like bad weather, blisters, or a run that just didn't go to plan to more considerable lows, such as an injury that stops you from running completely while you heal. As difficult as these times are, I firmly believe that the runner's highs will always outweigh the lows and there are ways to get through them all.

MANAGING SLIGHT INCONVENIENCES

Let's start with the easy ones: those little inconveniences that might make us feel like our run was below par, leave us a bit grumpy and perhaps feeling like we've been denied the joy of our run. I can think of a few things that have annoyed me on a run over the years, like wearing clothes that rub, a diversion on my route, forgetting my headphones or – on one recent occasion – almost losing one of my AirPods completely mid-run.

I was running on a windy day, listening to Bryony Gordon interviewing Jessica Ennis-Hill on her podcast, *Mad World*, and really enjoying it, when a branch suddenly flew out of nowhere and hit my ear. The AirPod flew out across the road and right underneath a parked car.

I knew this would happen one day! I thought, rolling my eyes.

They'd only play if both are in your ears, plus they're quite expensive, so leaving it wasn't an option. Moments later, there I was, lying on the pavement, grasping and stretching under the car, desperately trying to reach it. It was a bit embarrassing, and I'm sure I drew some strange looks, but guess what?

I got it back. I listened to the rest of the podcast and it was great.

I could have been annoyed at the weather for blowing a branch at my head and vow never to run in the wind again. I could focus on the embarrassment, or the disappointment that my run was slower because of the interruption. But positivity is how I choose to approach the small setbacks that running throws at you. Rather than dwell on negative emotions, I try to reframe them in a positive manner.

Forgotten your headphones so you can't catch up on your podcasts? No worries, you can listen to the birds singing in the park instead – how lovely is that?

Is a road closed on your usual route, so you've been forced to take a different way home? Well, how exciting! You've never run that way before, what might you find? Will you get a bit more distance in, or maybe get home faster?

Tripped over in a race? Thank goodness it wasn't worse – and how nice was it that the runner behind you stopped to pick you up?

Faithful trainers giving you blisters? Thank them for their service and start shopping – new trainers are always a treat!

About to go on your run, but the rain is torrential? Don't worry, your skin is waterproof! Once you get started, you'll be fine – and just think how good that hot shower is going to feel when you get back.

Returning to the scene of a bad run? Don't dwell on the negatives. Push out those bad memories and reinforce the good. I tend to remind myself things like: 'This is the bit where I always see those gorgeous birds flying', 'This is where I always overtake the bus. I love it because I'm faster than the traffic here'.

Can't shake off feeling rubbish on a run? Smile and tell yourself 'I love this bit' even if you don't 100 per cent mean it. You see, smiling – whether genuine or not – releases your feelgood hormones, dopamine, endorphins and serotonin. These send a signal to your body that you're happy and in turn, you do actually start to feel happier. Magic, eh?

A positive mindset is such a powerful tool in getting past the small annoyances and difficulties we face when running, but equally important is not dwelling on things that haven't gone to plan. My mum always says that when something goes wrong, put it behind you. It's done, you can't change it, so move on. And do you know what? She's absolutely right.

BLISTERS, CHAFING, CRAMPS, STITCH AND TOENAIL TRAUMA

There are certain things in a runner's life that are something of a rite of passage. One of them is losing a toenail … or so I thought. I was hosting the TV coverage of the Brighton Marathon in 2014 and Paula Radcliffe was starting the race. Thinking I'd engage in a little runner-to-runner chat, I asked if she'd ever lost a toenail.

'No, I've never lost one,' she said.

Well, that killed the conversation. I'd lost loads and had assumed it was something of a dubious badge of honour. All I could think was, *What am I doing wrong?*

The process of losing a toenail is grim. First, it goes purply black, like a bruise under the nail. Then the nail becomes loose and starts to peel away from the toe until you can just pull it away – gross!

Apparently though, you can avoid losing them in the first place. You lose toenails when your shoes aren't properly fitted for running. They should be a size bigger than your normal. Oh, and remember to trim long toenails short.

I tend to wear a shoe half a size bigger – and that's why, as it stands, I have two missing toenails on each foot. Take heed, people!

Blisters

As I have mentioned earlier in this book, these are something we all face from the start, due to skin being damaged by friction and heat. They're horrible and they can completely ruin a run.

Now, if you are susceptible to blisters – and I used to be – every run, no matter how short, you should get the Vaseline pot out, take a big scoop and smear it on your feet. I used to do this as part of my routine. Vaseline on, I'd then put my socks and trainers on. It felt weird and made a real squelching, grim sound, but it would help me to avoid blisters. If you end up with a blister and it has slightly popped, then it could rub and the skin will come off. This will hurt and possibly ruin your run, so why not put a Compeed specialist blister plaster on it? Fabric plasters don't stay in place in the same way – they move around, roll up and end up rubbing you more. Compeed are much thicker and make running with a blister or sore much easier.

Cramp

I'm so lucky that I have never suffered from cramps when running, but I have witnessed someone else suffering from it and it looks agonising. I remember watching as their muscles moved around under the skin like something out of *Alien*.

Cramp can be caused by dehydration and electrolyte imbalances, but in the calf – where it is common for runners to experience it – it is because the glutes, hamstrings and calves aren't strong enough, which causes the muscles to spasm when they are worked hard[17].

Instead of running through a calf cramp, stop and stretch it out instead. Try a Downward Dog pose, putting the weight of the body on the palms and the feet, arms are stretched straight forward, shoulder width apart, head down and pointing towards the floor. The feet should be about a foot apart, legs are straight, and the hips raised as high as possible. Or alternatively, do standing bent-over toe touches until you feel ready to try running again and incorporate calve-strengthening exercises into your strength and conditioning sessions. Stay well-hydrated too.

Stitches

The dreaded stitch is a huge irritation and will affect all runners at some point. Although the exact cause of side stitches in running has yet to be proven, theories abound, including tension in the diaphragm, cramping in the abdominal muscles and irritation of structures within the abdominal cavity.

If you do find yourself with a stitch you should reduce your pace to a slow jog or even a walk, and gently push your hands into the area of discomfort, just under your ribs, to help ease the cramping. Try changing your breathing pattern for a few breaths too, taking a very deep breath in, then exhaling sharply.

Chafing

Thighs, nipples, armpits and the groin are all areas where most runners have experienced some form of chafing or another. Caused when skin rubs against skin or clothing, it can leave a painful and even a bloody rash and makes your post-run shower or ice bath extremely uncomfortable (not to mention walking or running in the days that follow).

To avoid chafing, pick clothes that fit, avoid or remove tags or labels that might rub you and cover yourself in anti-chafe cream. Vaseline is the cheap and effective classic of course (and it's why you see it lined up on sticks at marathons, ready for runners to top up) but there are plenty of options to explore.

As most women wear bras, we tend to escape the horror of 'runner's nipple', but men may want to consider a nipple cover to prevent chafing in this area, this can be in the form of circular adhesive tape, a bandage or even lubricating ointment. Prevention really is key, but if you do get caught out, here's how to deal with the issue:

1. Clean the area to remove sweat, dirt and bacteria

2. Gently pat it dry

3. Apply an antibacterial cream – you can't go wrong with Sudocrem

4. Put loose clothes on and allow your skin to heal.

TOILET TROUBLES

Now, needing a pee when you're out on a run is one thing but there's nothing worse than the horror of sudden cramps in your stomach and an urgent dash to find a loo when an attack of the 'runner's trots' (runner's diarrhoea) kicks in. I bet anyone reading this who has run more than a few kilometres in one go is nodding in agreement here. One minute, you're fine and happily running along, then suddenly it will hit you out of the blue – the gurgle, the sharp cramp. You know exactly what it means …

I need to go, and I need to go now!

Inevitably, you'll be quite a distance from home so the panic sets in. Cold sweat forms on your forehead and you start clutching your stomach. You look around and there's no public loo in sight.

Oh my God, what am I going to do? you think.

You may, as I have, had to go somewhere like a gym and beg them to use the loo, even though you're not a member. You might find some resistance, but I found that standing in their foyer, sweating, clutching my tummy and saying, 'I WILL have an accident right here in about ten seconds if I don't get to the loo' worked a treat! You might even have had to crouch on the ground, taking deep breaths and willing the sensation to pass. Sometimes you're lucky and it does. Then you just have to run home and hope for the best.

It's not just the inconvenience, embarrassment and the pain of the situation either. If it happens on a Race Day, having to find a loo or being slowed down by debilitating cramps can derail a PB or leave you in agony mid-race. In fact, it doesn't matter who you are, how experienced you are, runner's trots can affect anyone, even elite runners – when you've got to go, you've got to go!

WHAT CAUSES RUNNER'S TROTS?

There isn't one definitive cause for runner's trots, there are lots of factors but here are some of the most common.

The mechanics of the body – The movement of your body and organs as you run can make you need to poop. The upper gastrointestinal (GI) tract moves more, so the likelihood of a bowel movement is increased.

Dehydration and low electrolytes – If you lose fluid in your body and don't replace it fast enough, this can cause diarrhoea. A particular risk for runners who have not pre-hydrated enough ahead of a longer run.

Eating too much and too close to a run – When you run, all the blood flow is directed to your muscles to help you move, so the stomach can't digest food as normal. When that happens and your stomach is full, it can cause diarrhoea.

Not eating enough – Don't be tempted to try and avoid runner's trots by not eating before a run. Either not fuelling properly for a run, or not eating enough in general can cause 'leaky gut', which will in turn cause tummy upsets and loose bowel movements.

Too much fibre – Eating too much fibrous foods like beans, fruit and salad can trigger runner's diarrhoea.

Unfamiliar foods and supplements – Trying new gels, chews or eating foods you don't usually eat risks giving you an upset stomach and diarrhoea. High-fibre, high-fat foods, sweeteners or caffeine can all be a factor too. Also, taking any gels too fast can mean the glucose hit to your stomach is too intense and might give you the urge to, you know, *go …*

Pre-race nerves – If you're feeling jittery about a race, the stress and anxiety can have an impact on your gut too.

DEALING WITH RUNNER'S TROTS

When it comes to dealing with runner's trots, there are things you can do to minimise the chance of them happening and measures you can put in place to ensure you're prepared if you are caught out. To minimise your chances:

* Avoid eating fibre-rich food before a long run or race (my pre-long run snack is a dry bagel!).

* Make sure you're well hydrated and stay that way as you run.

* Eat something before your run – exactly when is a very individual choice and there are no rules. I personally tend not to run too soon after eating in case I get a stitch or need to stop for the loo, but it really is a case of try and test.

* Don't try new foods or gels on Race Day in case they upset your stomach.

* Consume gels gradually (over five minutes). Apparently, you shouldn't take them too fast because the intense glucose hit can make you want to go!

To manage the trots if you're caught out:

* On a general run, plan your route and know where the loos are – my routes go via McDonald's, cafés and park

toilets just in case (make sure you have change if you need to pay for a public loo). This works for frequent wee-ers too.

* Dehydration and low electrolytes can cause the trots, so during a race you can take some electrolytes by adding some powder or tablets to your water and sip it as you run.

* Take tissues/wipes – because portable loos and public toilets aren't always well stocked!

Fellas, please don't stop reading here – the next bit is for all genders!

PERIODS, PREGNANCY, MENOPAUSE AND MORE

Many of the challenges that we face as runners are universal, but let's be honest, fellas, you do have it a little easier! Due to our biology, hormones and physiological responses, there are things that set us females apart – periods, pregnancy, menopause – and times in our lives when we will find running more of a challenge, in ways that you won't.

You lucky things!

But just because it might not affect you directly, that doesn't mean you should skip this bit. If you run with your partner, sister, friend who happens to be a girl or if any of your running buddies might be affected by these challenges, the following sections could provide some useful insights.

RUNNING AND PREGNANCY

Now, I'm not for one second saying that getting pregnant is a low. Not at all, it's amazing, special and something that lots of us wait a long time for. But as a runner, it can throw up some challenges that can be quite difficult to navigate, which is why I'm talking about it here in this chapter.

I found out that I was pregnant in January 2010. At the time I was training hard and getting faster. In 2009, I ran a forty-two-minute 10K and even hit a marathon PB of 3 hours 35 minutes. I was running five times a week, I had a great strength training coach I was going to twice a week and I was enjoying living my life too, going out, eating and drinking as I pleased, and I was genuinely so happy. I had my eye on my next goals, a 3.15 marathon and a sub-1.30 half marathon and training was going well … until New Year's Day when I went out for one of my fifteen-mile training runs.

James and I had planned to meet friends for a pub lunch, so I'd timed it in such a way that I had enough time to get home and get ready. I started running my route, but when I got to Richmond Park, something just felt different:

I was out of breath in a way that I never had been before. I had to keep stopping and I just couldn't get my pace up so I rang James.

'You're going to have to come and get me,' I said.

'What?' he gasped.

I understood his surprise – I'm not sure I'd ever called him to pick me up from a run before.

'It's so weird, I'm just out of breath. I can't do it,' I said.

Of course, he came and got me, and we made it to the pub on time, but something was niggling. I was the absolute fittest I had ever been in my life. I wasn't ill, I wasn't tired. There was no reason at all for me to be out of breath. Nothing obvious had changed that might make me feel like this.

Unless …

I wonder if I'm pregnant …

The idea was plausible and it was the only thing I could think that might be different.

I spent the whole lunch with the thought spinning in my mind. As soon as I got home, I did a pregnancy test and my suspicion was confirmed: I was a few weeks pregnant. We were both over the moon, but this was my first baby and I had questions. What did me being pregnant mean for my running? I knew my 3 hours 15 marathon would be out of the window, but how far could I run? Would I even be able to run at all?

I was so used to hearing people say that you shouldn't

do anything, just sit there, rest and enjoy eating for two. The eating bit sounded good and I knew that at some point I physically wouldn't be able to run, but the idea of not doing the thing that I loved so much for nine months filled me with horror. I deferred my marathon to the April of the following year and I wasn't going to push myself, but I still wanted to be able to run so I consulted my GP.

'You can keep running,' she said.

'But how long can I run for?' I asked.

'It's more about how fast or hard you run,' she explained. 'You can only run at a pace that you are able to talk at. You must be able to keep your heart rate under control and you need to be able to breathe properly.'

Now that made perfect sense and I knew I could manage it.

'That's fine,' I said.

To make sure I ran at an easy pace, I would keep checking my ability to talk by chatting to myself (stopping whenever I passed someone, just so I didn't look too crazy!). I knew that if I could hold a full, normal conversation, I wasn't out of breath or anywhere near it.

Twice a week I went to the gym and would treat myself to some lovely carrot cake from the bakery on the way home. I kept on training and running more or less as usual with some simple adaptations all the way through.

When my little bump popped, about five or six months in, I found myself running with my leggings pulled under the bump and a normal top stretched over it, because at the time there wasn't anything in the way of running maternity gear. I looked like I had a beer gut poking out and as I ran, I could feel it swinging in the wind.

It felt super weird.

By six months, my body had completely changed and much as it shocked me to say it, I was done with running – it had just become too uncomfortable. But I still wanted to stay active, so I switched to the ski machine in the gym. I did that right up until my due date. By then my thighs were touching from the knee up and any kind of exercise was just too difficult to manage.

Time to stop.

Ella was born at the end of September, a week later than expected.

My mind went straight back to running. I had seven months until my deferred London Marathon.

I'm going to do this, I thought.

I was so excited to be a mum and I loved that bonding period with Ella, but I was still super focused on my marathon and I wanted to get started straight away. I had a mountain buggy pram you could run with, a plan and two weeks after the birth, I set out excitedly for my first run. But it felt completely weird. My knees felt like those bendy plastic rulers from school and with every step, they bent backwards and I started to worry they might snap. So I spoke to my GP to find out what was going on.

I didn't realise that when you have a baby and you're breastfeeding, you have a hormone called Relaxin produced by the ovaries and placenta in your body, which loosens and relaxes your joints, muscles and ligaments. It's great for childbirth and new motherhood, but terrible for running, especially since I was already hypermobile. It was causing my knees to overextend and I was at risk of causing a serious injury. On seeking advice from my GP, they told me my body just wasn't ready to run yet.

New mums weren't recommended to start strenuous exercise until at least six weeks after the birth, it transpired.

Throughout the whole of my pregnancy, I'd managed how I felt about not being able to run like I usually do. I'd even coped with not running at all in the last few months but that's because I had planned to be running and to be back training straight away. Though frustrating, I recognised that I had to reset my expectations.

It was a slower process than I'd hoped, but I started out by walking all the time. Then, after a couple of months, I was able to begin running again, starting with a few short treadmill jogs. It was January before I could run much further and having a newborn meant that I had to rework my running routine all over again – I had to make things work around my job, James's work and of course, Ella's routines.

I started off in the gym near our house, parking Ella in the pram next to the treadmill, where I essentially taught myself how to run again. When Ella was six months old, I was able to start running with her in the pram, which was a revelation. I could be a mum, run, walk the dog and pop to the shop for milk if needed – all at the same time! Walks with the dog would be a bit of a run/walk session, enforced intervals, as I'd have to stop for them going to the toilet. I did my long training runs in the gym on the treadmill, taking Ella in her pram when she was asleep and leaving when she woke up.

Now, fellas, I understand how becoming a dad is a huge, life-changing thing for you as well. It means completely adapting your running routine to fit in with a baby's schedule and of course supporting your partner – and my goodness, you're going to have some slow, tired jogs! It goes without saying that it's important to communicate with your other half about how things are for you, but also for you to understand what she's going through – that way, you can work more effectively as a team and make sure everyone is happy, healthy (and getting their runs in!).

I was so lucky because James and I were a great team as we got used to the routine of having a baby. With him being a night owl, when Ella was ready for the bottle, he took most of the middle-of-the-night feeds and I did the early ones because I'd be up for work. Don't get me wrong, there were times when we were both exhausted because she was teething or whatever and we'd be so broken. I fell asleep in the make-up chair at *This Morning* multiple times, but looking back, it really was a very short period of time.

So, we managed it. We cracked being new parents and I managed to get back to doing the thing I loved – running. Just seven months after giving birth to our amazing Ella, I crossed the finish line of the London Marathon in three hours, fifty-one minutes. It wasn't my 3 hours 15. But after the complete change my body – and my entire life – had been through, sixteen minutes slower than my PB was all right with me!

MANAGING MENOPAUSE

For those of us who will experience menopause, it's a time in our lives when running might be more of a challenge. Due to the nature of the symptoms of menopause, particularly those who experience them more severely, it will likely impact those around you too so for that reason I think it's worth people of all genders knowing about the subject. Now this is super basic, so forgive me, but to get us all up to speed: According to the NHS Menopause generally happens to women between the ages of forty-five to fifty-five, with fifty-one being the average age for the onset of menopause. It is the result of changes in the level of the hormone oestrogen in the body. There are three specific stages:

Perimenopause – The time before menopause when symptoms (irregular periods, hot flushes, brain fog, mood swings, headaches, anxiety etc.) can present. Generally speaking, this can start up to ten years before the menopause.

Menopause – This is a specific moment, marking twelve consecutive months without a period.

Postmenopausal – The life stage after menopause when periods have stopped.

As coach and runner extraordinaire Karen Weir explained in a *RunPod* special, perimenopause is a time of 'chaos in the body' and whether we like it or not, it's going to have an impact on our running. We will get slower; our bodies will respond differently to the cortisol produced when we exercise. However, it's not a reason to stop. In fact, continuing to exercise is important to maintain your mental health through this stage in your life and ensure that your physical health means you have the best possible quality of life as you age.

Throughout our life, the hormones oestrogen and progesterone help us to adapt to the exercise that we do. They are the stimuli that help us to build muscle, improve cardiovascular health and much more. When oestrogen levels start to drop, we just need to learn how to adapt to those changing levels of hormones in our body. Now, this is a huge and complex topic that we couldn't possibly cover in full here and there are whole books dedicated just to this, such as *Next Level: Your Guide to Kicking Ass, Feeling Great, and Crushing Goals Through Menopause and Beyond* by Dr Stacy Sims, PhD, as recommended by Karen. But if you are approaching menopause (or are even still a way off it), there are a few things I would recommend:

Think ahead and take action that will help future you – For example, strength training as soon as possible, whether that be in your twenties or thirties, will help you improve bone density and build muscle. We lose both in menopause, so creating a good foundation early on will help you later and mean you're less at risk of conditions like osteoporosis which can weaken the bones meaning they could break more easily. You could also experience back pain which may give you a more stooped posture. But even if you are late to the game and have already gone through perimenopause or menopause, it is never too late to start weight-training and can only help you in the long term.

Run for your mental health – There are lots of brain-related menopause symptoms and anxiety and depression can be common. Continuing to run can help alleviate some of those symptoms.

Work hard but do less – Long runs and lots of reps in the gym will raise cortisol levels, which can exacerbate the symptoms of menopause, so you might need to change up how you train. You could still do long runs, but I would recommend mixing it up and maybe introducing more short, fast, sprint training, or interval sessions, as well as the weight training and plyometric sessions. Still get out for your long run if you want, however make sure that you complement these sessions with different workouts on other days.

Eat a balanced diet and prioritise protein – We start to lose muscle from the age of thirty and the loss increases during the perimenopause. Proteins are our body's building blocks, so at a time when even maintaining muscle is a challenge, we need it more than ever.

Consider supplementation – This is a time when women could experience one of dozens of symptoms from anxiety to sleepless nights, hot sweats to joint pain and also lack of motivation to exercise and sudden weight gain. These can make life even more challenging at a time when hormones are already fluctuating – supplements can be a way to manage these symptoms.

Incorporate strength training and plyometric training (jump training) – Both help maintain muscle and support bone strength, as well as helping to manage weight, cutting the risk of diseases such as diabetes, heart disease and stroke.

Adapt your training – You can still aim for a marathon, but if you try to train for it in the same way as you did at twenty or thirty, you'll end up fatigued and with injuries. Make sure your training supports where your body is now.

Re-evaluate your goals – The way your body needs you to train at this stage of your life might not be ideal for long-distance goals like marathons and ultramarathons, but you could be smashing PBs in those shorter distances. Why not focus your goals on 5 and 10K targets?

RUNNER'S NIGHTMARE: INJURY

OK, OK, so I said earlier that runner's trots were the worst, but I lied. The worst thing that can possibly happen to a runner is an injury that means they have to reduce – even completely stop – running. Unfortunately, it is also something we're unlikely to completely avoid. Some injuries will be minor and require a few days' rest but others take much more time to heal.

I speak from experience as I have had LOADS.

I fractured my foot at a terrible time. It was during

lockdown, when I was running almost every day (for my sanity even more than usual, like so many others who ran during the pandemic). It wasn't like breaking a leg – snap and I knew something had gone. Instead, my foot just swelled to an enormous size until I couldn't get a shoe on or do much more than hobble about. At the time hospitals were understandably overwhelmed by Covid patients, so it took six weeks for me to get an MRI scan and a diagnosis from a physio.

'It's a stress fracture,' they said.

In case you don't know, a stress fracture is a tiny crack in a bone, usually caused by repetitive force. Basically, I overdid it. I was sentenced to six weeks in a boot and I was devastated. I'd already gone without running for six weeks, the thought of another six weeks off horrified me. But I had no choice. No matter how amazing I'd felt while I'd been running seven or eight miles every day that led to the injury, I had to accept that my body was broken, I was knackered and I needed to recover.

While running too much had caused my injury, not running now presented me with another problem: I didn't just use running to stay fit and healthy. I used it to get perspective and clarity on life, organise my thoughts and manage my stress and anxiety. So, if I couldn't run, what could I do to fill that gap?

RANGAN'S STORY

The idea of having something to fall back on during injury came up in my *RunPod* chat with Dr Rangan Chatterjee, a doctor, presenter, runner and author of books including *Happy Mind, Happy Life*.

Talking in April 2022 about how he got into running and his experience of injury during the marathon, we discussed how many of us use running to escape and reflect on our lives, to release stress and find balance, which is great. But what if you can't run?

'I kind of feel that all of us at some point need to develop the skill of releasing stress without running as well,' he said. 'If running is your only release, then what happens when you get injured?

'It's so big and people really struggle. Their life starts to fall to pieces because they used to have this wonderful regime and routine with running, but suddenly their ankle's gone or their hamstring's gone and they have to rest for a few weeks,' he explained. 'Suddenly they get anxious, their mood goes, it affects their relationships. So, I think it's a good skill for people to learn a non-moving form of relaxation and perspective-taking too. That could be journalling, meditation on an app like Calm or Headspace – just don't put all your eggs in one basket. I would just encourage people to think about it. Is there anything else I can bring in as well that means, should something happen where I can't run, I still have something to help me unwind and de-stress?'

To illustrate his point, Rangan shared the story of one of his clients, a runner who, through injury, found herself not just unable to run, but unable to walk or even leave the house.

'Running was her release, it was how she unwound, it was how she dealt with the stress of work; but she got injured. She couldn't walk, she couldn't leave the house,' he said. 'I taught her how to journal and it was transformative for her. Before that she had two weeks of absolute hell and then she started journalling every morning, with her morning cup of coffee.

'She was just writing down anything that was coming into her mind and she told me: "When I run, I process certain thoughts, but journalling has processed my thoughts a slightly different way, so I have learnt different things about myself and my life in a way I don't when I'm running,"' he explained. 'I'm always keen to make people bulletproof, so that no matter what happens in life, they've got options of where to turn to.'

FINDING YOUR FALLBACK

I completely related to what Rangan said about how runners' moods change when they can't run and the profound effect it can have on your mental health. When I can't run, I absolutely hate it. Thankfully, when I found myself stuck in a boot with my stress fracture, I didn't need to find a non-moving alternative to running as Rangan suggested, as I was lucky that I was still able to get around, albeit a bit lopsided and uneven. And fortunately for me (and my family), I was able to turn to another hobby, which gave me a little bit of the same release and balance that running gave me – playing golf. And my goodness, did I love being able to focus on it!

Playing golf is a different kind of high, so I missed running, of course. But I loved being able to still play another sport I truly love, even in a boot. The only thing is I had to use a golf buggy, so it was hardly the most cardio of workouts. Even so, the fact that you have to focus still allowed me to escape for a few hours and zone out away from the world of emails and technology. It's also hugely social whereas when I run, I usually run alone. So, it might not be sitting still, but Rangan, if you're reading this, it was the closest I was going to get!

WHAT CAUSES INJURY AND HOW TO AVOID IT

Now, once you've been injured and it's taken you away from something you love, you do become much more aware of what your body is telling you. In the summer of 2022, I was training hard for the London Marathon. I was on holiday in Spain with Ella and James, but getting up at the break of dawn to do my seventeen-mile training runs before the heat of the day set in.

I hadn't run intensively for a while, having had several injuries and just an increasingly busy schedule, but now I was running five times a week. While I was training, I noticed something was wrong in my hip area. Even if I slowed down to walk it was really, really sore and it looked swollen too. In fact, on holiday my hips became so swollen, you might have thought I'd had hip and butt implants – but only on my left side! Eventually by the time I returned from holiday, the pain got so bad, I went to the physio and they ended up sending me for an MRI scan. Turns out that I had a torn Iliotibial (IT) band, the tendon that runs along the outside of your leg, which can tear if it's placed under excessive stress, and gluteal tendinopathy, pain around the outside of the hip as a result of frequent compression of the tendons over a period of time.

Once again there was nothing for it apart from rest, rehabilitation and hanging up my trainers for four months.

Realising that I'd have to withdraw from the marathon, I was heartbroken.

Four months was a long time but the risk of extending that time by being daft and trying to get going again too soon would be even more annoying and frustrating. I had to be sensible. Sometimes you have to step away and get strong in order to come back sooner, so that is what I did.

I knew that I would be able to run again, and the break was good. It gave me time to really focus on strength work, which I had regretfully neglected for too long and was probably a factor in why I got injured in the first place. Mike Gornall, my brilliant PT at CrossFit Putney, had me doing exercises that would strengthen the areas that needed attention – my back, core, legs and glutes. All going to plan, I would be ready to run again in a few months. In the meantime, as well as getting stronger in the gym, I got better at golf too, so it was actually a productive few months.

I also reminded myself that when I was able to start back, I'd be like a new runner again, building myself back up and experiencing all the joy and enjoyment of that once again.

When I was able to run again, oh, my goodness, I was on top of the world, my smile beaming every time I went out the door. The break reminded me that there are so many people who can't run permanently, who are desperate to get out there, and I just felt so lucky.

AVOIDING INJURY

According to Bupa private healthcare, sport injuries in general are divided into four categories:

* Overuse (training hard and not giving your body enough time to recover)
* Trauma (falls and collisions)
* Fractures and dislocations
* Sprains and strains (ligament and muscle injuries).

Most running injuries apparently fall into the overuse category, something that does not surprise me in the slightest, given that this (and a few pairs of ill-fitting trainers!) have been the cause of most of mine. You see, we runners love running. Most of us would run every day if our bodies and schedules would allow, to feel the elation and high that it gives us and help us work towards our goals. But to be able to enjoy the sport for a long time, we must find the balance, which is why I focus on the following to do my best to avoid new injuries (or aggravating old ones):

1. Don't run every single day of the week, allow for rest – I currently run four to five times per week, with a couple of rest days.

2. Wear shoes that fit you – I don't think I can ever say this enough. Ill-fitting shoes will end in injury!

3. Include strength, conditioning and flexibility exercises in your training routine – I've suggested the ones I use in Chapter 5 (see also pages 125–35).

4. Listen to your body – If there's a persistent niggle, get it checked out by a GP or physio. You could be making it worse if you keep pushing.

5. Build up gradually – Pushing for a new time or distance? Don't try and do it too quickly, work up in stages so you don't put your body under too much stress.

6. If you're told to stop running, stop – As devastating and frustrating as it is, listen to the experts. If you don't, you could end up out of action a hell of a lot longer.

7. Focus on recovery – I have recently been inducted into the ice bath gang and I love it! Lots of runners swear by an ice-bath post-run to promote recovery and loosen stiff muscles. There's a variety of options, but the small, inflatable types are popular and very affordable. You can also use handheld massagers to relieve sore muscles or book a good sports massage.

8. Develop strategies for managing your mental health when you can't run – For me, it's golf and walking. For you, it might be journalling or meditation. Where possible, make sure you know what your fallback is *before* you're injured.

8

THE POWER OF COMMUNITY

There's a famous moment from the 2017 London Marathon, which saw Matthew Rees, a member of the Swansea Harriers running club, walk fellow runner, David Wyeth, from Chorlton Runners, over the finish line, arm in arm. About 300 metres from the end of the race, Matthew was about to sprint to the finish line when David staggered in front of him, legs like jelly, and collapsed. David was a complete stranger, but in that moment, Matthew made the decision to forget his own race.

Cameras captured the footage of him holding a staggering David up and helping him to the finish line and beamed it around the world.

These two men did not know each other at all, so what had compelled Matthew to abandon his own race to ensure David finished his? After the race, Matthew explained: 'He had come so far and after twenty-six miles of running, I wanted him to make the finish.'

It's moments like this that perfectly demonstrate the true nature of the running community. United by a mutual passion for running, an understanding of what it takes to push yourself to your limits and more than anything, just wanting one another to succeed. The story hit the headlines and even prompted the creation of a special Spirit of the London Marathon award, which celebrates people and moments that embody that attitude that's at the heart of the race.

For me, the spirit of the London Marathon is the spirit of the running community as a whole. It just holds a big, beautiful mirror up to it. As Matthew himself pointed out in interviews and appearances that followed, acts of kindness and support like his happen all the time in the running community – they're just not always caught on camera.

More recently, at the 2023 Great North Run, a 102-year-old World War II veteran became the oldest person ever to finish a half marathon. William 'Bill' Cooksey took on the challenge to raise money for County Durham and Darlington NHS Trust and completed the 13.1-mile course in five hours and forty-one minutes, aided by his friend, Gavin Iceton. He crossed the finish line to enormous applause from crowds, who had waited in heavy rain just to celebrate his achievement.

Moments like this one, and Matthew Rees' display of sportsmanship, happen because the running community – those who participate and those who support – is so unified in its love for the sport and its mutual admiration and respect for all who take part, regardless of level or ability. It's a bond that starts from the minute you run out of your door.

IT STARTS WITH 'RUNNING BUDDIES'

Every day for years, as I run home from work along the river, I see the same man with his little dog at least three times a week. We pass one another, nod, smile and carry on. One day I decided that I saw him so often, I really should say something. So, the next time I saw him, I stopped him.

'I have to say hello,' I said. 'I see you every morning.'

'And I listen to you every day on Smooth,' he told me. 'When I hear you say goodbye on air, I know it won't be long before I see you!'

His name is Dennis and he's now what I class as one of my 'running buddies'. It's a connection that exists for no other reason than the fact that I happen to regularly run past him. We'll sometimes stop and have a little chat, and it's lovely.

The running community is built on the foundation of interactions like this. It's a special and immediate bond that all runners and those who interact with them share. A bond that's particularly strong when you're *both* runners. I could meet you and strike up a conversation: You're running, I'm running, and we both get stuck at the traffic lights, crossing the road. I won't ask you your name, I won't ask you what you do for a living, I won't ask you where you're from. But I'll probably say: 'How's your run?' or 'Nice trainers, where are they from?'

We'll have a really great, short chat about running and I know that I'll take more away from that than I would other small talk about what you do for a living or where you're from, because none of that other stuff matters when you're chatting about running – the topic acts as a leveller. That's why running is so brilliant, because it brings and binds people together over a common interest, with no prejudices and no judgement.

One of the first times I *really* noticed this about running was after a run I had been invited to that had been organised by a new app to specifically introduce runners to one another. There were loads of people, some I recognised from 'running Instagram' but others I didn't know at all. We did a 5K run around a park near Tooting in South London, then we all went on to the pub for a drink and carried on chatting for ages – about running, of course. That was literally all we talked about, for hours and hours. And despite what any non-runner might think, it was a really fun evening.

I remember looking around at one point and thinking how incredible it was that we were all so different. In terms of backgrounds, jobs, everything. Our ages were varied, some had kids, others were singletons. We had fast and slow runners. Some were outgoing, others were quiet, each of us was totally unique. In fact, I'd go as far as to say that we were all so different that without that event, perhaps most of us would never have met, let alone been chatting like old friends in that pub. But despite our obvious differences there was no division in the group, no elitism – for we all had one thing in common – we were all runners and the conversation never once ran out. I'm still friends with many of those people today, along with the people I've met nervously at start lines, lurching across finish lines and just jogging around wherever I find myself.

The running community makes itself known to you as soon as you start to run. It starts with a nod to a fellow runner, develops into a chat with another jogger when you're stopped at the traffic lights and it's cemented when you look forward to catching up with your fellow parkrunners on a Saturday morning.

When you run, you immediately belong.

FINDING YOUR RUNNING TRIBE

While runners are one big happy family, the running community also has many different parts and exists in a variety of forms. From solo runners who share progress online and weekly fun run meetups, to virtual communities and local running clubs – we all have to find our own running tribe. Consider why you run, what you want to achieve and what you enjoy about running, and you'll soon find the corner of the running community where your people exist!

Run for fun and want to make friends? Find no-pressure socially-focused running groups that fit your own interests – there's parkrun, pub runs and other runs that involve stopping for coffee and cake, yum!

New or returning to running? Find a local non-competitive group with a coach who can help and support you to achieve your goals, whether that's 0 to 5K, or just getting out a few times a week.

Training for races or wanting to push your limits? More traditional, competitive running clubs might suit you as you can learn from peers, coaches and run leads. They will know where all the good races are, so you can get involved and there are even groups that specifically focus on big challenges and ultramarathons.

Want to escape the city and run in the hills and forests?
Find a trail running group to run and explore with or check
out the Love Trails Festival, where you can run, dance, wild
swim, adventure and party in the Gower Peninsula in Wales.

**Want to meet more people who are into running and go
from there?** Not ready to run with others yet? Want to
chat and learn more first? Why not start off volunteering?
You could be a marshal at a fun run or help out at a local
parkrun. Get chatting to other runners and volunteers and
see where they run. You might form your perfect group
that way, or just make friends who you can run with!

FORGET THE 118 118 MEN

When I first started running, I was enormously intimidated
by the thought of joining a running club. It was a scary
prospect, because it was full of professional runners, right?
For those of us old enough to remember the campaign
that launched 118 118 directory enquiries in 2002, I was
convinced that running clubs would be full of super enthu-
siastic people dressed like the iconic athletic-vest and
short-shorts wearing men in the TV adverts, who sprinted
around, shouting, 'Got your number!'

I wasn't professional, I ran for fun. So, I thought that they
weren't for me.

It was only much later that I learnt I was completely wrong about running clubs. Yes, there are clubs that are more suited to those aiming for big races, faster times and being competitive. But that didn't mean they were aloof or unrelatable, far from it. In fact, they provide a community of people who will motivate you, advise and help you to progress and achieve your goals. As I've said before, runners have one another's backs, even when you're at different points in your journey. But as well as those – the 'traditional' running clubs – there are literally THOUSANDS of other running clubs and groups around the UK that are focused on different things, like the social aspect of running together, or particular styles of running. Whatever you're looking for, there will be one for you. Here's a few types that you can look out for in your area.

parkrun – No discussion about the running community would be complete without a mention of parkrun. So many people start going just to get fit and end up falling completely in love with running and making new friends. Established as we know it today in 2008, its founder Paul Sinton-Hewitt, a club runner, marathoner and indeed past *RunPod* guest, actually first set up the event in Bushy Park in the London borough of Richmond-upon-Thames in 2004, after sustaining a serious injury.

Suffering from depression and unable to run (the

way he would usually tackle low times), Paul started the regular event because he wanted to continue to spend time with his running friends and others interested in the pastime. He offered to manage a free, weekly, timed run to anyone who would like to attend, saying: 'The only condition was that they stay afterwards and go for coffee with me' – he credits the event with helping him out of his depression.

At the time of writing there are 800 parkrun locations in the UK. There are free weekly community 5Ks each Saturday and junior parkrun for four- to fourteen-year-olds, a 2K event each Sunday. It's a lovely way to experience community and running alongside other runners – a little first dip in for many people. Go to a parkrun and you will find people of your ability, and you'll cross a finish line at the same time.

Spectators and volunteers are also a key part of the parkrun community and it's a completely inclusive event – you can walk or run (or a combination), there is no time limit and parkrun signage, markers and finish line remain out until everyone completes the course. There is no 'last place', thanks to an army of volunteer tail walkers who make sure that no one is left behind.

You'll find your people running whether you're slow at the back, fast at the front or in the middle. You'll find your age group, you'll find everything … There's the chat before and often there's tea and coffee afterwards too. The more you go, the longer you'll stay and chat at the end, and you may find new friends and allies.

You can also go to parkruns away from your local area, be a 'tourist' as they call it. OK, you might not make friends for life there, but it gives you a ready-made community when you're travelling or working away, you can experience running in other places and you'll probably end up following some of the people you meet on socials too, widening your running network.

Traditional running clubs – These will usually be more established groups and may even have members who are professional runners, and there will usually be a membership fee to join. But despite looking a bit scary, they are still extremely friendly, welcoming places and will have groups for all abilities, so don't think it's not a place for you.

Local running groups – These may be more informal than traditional running clubs and might be led by one or a group of run leaders. Some will be free, others may require a small contribution to participate. Sometimes running groups will be established around a common factor, like buggy running groups for new mums, LGBT+ focused running groups or groups that have a strong social aspect, like early-morning runs ending with a hearty breakfast at a local café.

Branded running groups – Sports organisations some-times establish running initiatives that are rolled out across the country, so there might be a group near you. For example, the RunTogether initiative from England Athletics has more than 2,000 groups across the country and offers a range of options from walk-jog sessions to more challenging runs.

Community action groups – There are some running groups that combine a good run with doing good for the local community. For example, GoodGym has groups all over England that 'get fit by doing good'. They run (and walk and cycle) while doing tasks to help others, such as litter picking, shifting earth for community gardens and delivering prescriptions to isolated older people. Good for the body, heart and soul!

Try the following websites or search on social media for your local parkrun, or running groups and clubs near you:

blackgirlsdorun.co.uk
englandathletics.org/find-a-club/
goodgym.org/
goodrunguide.co.uk/ClubFinder.asp
jogscotland.org.uk
meetup.com/topics/running/gb/
parkrun.org.uk/
rundemcrew.com/

runtalkrun.com/
runtogether.co.uk
thisgirlruns.club/find-a-club/

Some other good places to find out what running communities exist near you are at your local running store (when you go in for some new kit, why not ask one of the store assistants what's happening locally? They'll be bound to know), or ask about running groups at your gym.

ONLINE COMMUNITIES

While in-person groups are the foundation of our community, the internet and social media has done so much to bring it even closer together, connecting runners around the world and even recruiting many more to our numbers.

How many people have got hooked into running by seeing runners on social media and being inspired to get out there by their sweaty, smiley end-of-run selfies? If you're already a runner, this is the kind of content you want to see, because it motivates and inspires you. Our community online is what helps us flourish offline.

When I went out running, I could listen to music but sometimes I fancied listening to a podcast. I tried comedy podcasts and interviews, and they were great, but I wanted something that encouraged me to keep running. So that's how *RunPod* was born. It was 2018 and I was running home from my radio show when I thought, *what if I was listening to people chat about the feel good factor of running?* By hearing others share their reason to run, surely it would remind me of why I was out there pounding the pavements? Maybe, at times when I might want to stop, I'd hear guests say 'keep going' and I'd be encouraged to run a little further or faster?

RunPod came out in 2019 and was a success. I was not only proud that people actually listened to each episode, but that many did so while out running – to this day they still do. The listeners have become an amazing community of runners – old, new, fast, slow – and together we are The *RunPod* Run Club! We even have a Facebook group of the same name, where thousands of listeners are now members and part of a special group where there is only positive and supportive chat, all centred around running.

I was surprised by how it took off. Almost immediately, the group had 2,000 members. Today it has around 6,000 and that number grows every week. Just like that group in the pub, there are so many different people, at different running levels, but none of those differences matter. They all just look out for each other, a circle of virtual friends.

I'm so proud of how positive and welcoming a space it is and it's been so lovely to see people supporting one another in running and life challenges, providing accountability, motivating, inspiring, sharing advice, seeing them hit PBs and take on 5K, 10K, marathons and more.

But The *RunPod* Run Club isn't the only online community out there. There are LOADS, such as This Mum Runs, an online community of more than 200,000 that aims to connect women (not *just* mums), encourage them to put their wellbeing back at the top of the to-do list and get out running, the Slow AF Run Club, which connects the 'back of the pack' slow runners and walkers of the world and helps them to achieve their goals, and Lonely Goat, a huge online community that encourages members to support each other along their varied paths, celebrate ALL achievements and unites them through a sense of identity, common purpose and belonging. As well as providing a constant source of support and a ready-made army of cheerleaders, there are some other ways that the digital world has bolstered and enhanced the running community …

Strava (and other apps) – Billed as 'the social network for athletes', Strava is used by 100 million people in 195 countries – and runners make up a considerable proportion. First of all, I LOVE that every user in this community is considered 'an athlete'. As well as using it to track your runs and connect with friends, it's also a great way to engage with the wider running community. You can share your routes and photos and find new places to run by looking at routes that other runners have posted. You can take part in running challenges and try and make it onto a leader board, leave comments or give 'Kudos' to others for their runs, virtually congratulating them on their achievements.

There are of course lots of apps that runners use to track, and share runs, get involved in challenges and connect with friends. Some of the better-known ones are backed by major sports brands like Under Armour's MapMyRun, the Nike Run Club app or Runkeeper, which was acquired by ASICS, so it's worth taking some time to explore what's out there. Regardless of which you choose, the thing that makes them all brilliant is that even when we might not be physically connected, they reflect all the best elements of the running community: the human interaction, the inspiration and cheerleading, the celebration of success and lifting one another up.

Virtual races – Virtual races work just like any normal race – the only thing is you can do it anywhere: from your local park to a treadmill in the gym, or even abroad. All you have to do is provide evidence that you completed it, so you can get your medal or certificate.

You can run a virtual race for fun, to compete with a friend or for a charitable cause – it really is up to you. If you're part of a big online community that can't meet in person, virtual runs might be a great way to come together for the same challenge, from wherever each member may be.

You can find all kinds of virtual races and lots of major races now also have virtual spin-offs, like the TCS London Marathon MyWay, which allows you to complete 26.2 miles however and wherever you wish on Marathon Day, so even if you can't get to a race, you can still get involved.

RACES

Now parkrun, running groups and virtual communities are great, but you haven't experienced the running community until you've attended a race. You don't even have to run if you're not ready (although I highly recommend that you do), you can attend one or even volunteer, just to experience the atmosphere. If you don't run that time, I guarantee what you see and feel will have you signing up for the next race!

Now, despite the fact that I started running in 1995, I didn't run my first race until 2006. I was motivated enough to do all the runs, but I thought I wasn't good enough to qualify or even be able to consider doing any kind of race. I thought that races were just for people who were super-hot at running and I didn't see it as an inclusive thing. But the more I talked publicly about my love of running, the more people kept asking: 'Why don't you do a race?'

'Ha, I can't run that! I run for fun, I'm not serious,' I'd reply.

Because the thing is, I didn't think you could be both.

I didn't think you could do a race and just enjoy running – I thought if you do a race, you had to be in it to win it.

Eventually though, I got convinced to give one a go. The 2006 Nike 10K Run London: North vs South event was happening in London's Hyde Park and they offered me and my friend and GMTV co-presenter Ben Shephard a place. Our agent George Ashton also got a spot, so the three of us headed off to the start line. It was a new race that basically pitted North Londoners against South Londoners in Central London – 'two teams, one 10K' was the strapline. You signed up for the side of the city you wanted to run for, got your team shirt – green for North and orange for South – and you ran for your team. George and I were team South, Ben was team North.

Waiting at the start line, I was terrified. What an earth had I got into? Momentarily I felt like I must be the most under-qualified person there but then I realised that everyone was nervous, aware that we were all about to run a race. It was exciting and we were all excited about the same thing. The camaraderie was lovely, with people smiling and chatting, until the starter called out for our attention.

Ten, 9, 8 … we all counted down.

As the countdown reached one and the starting gun went, everyone clicked their watches and we were off! The buzz, the excitement, the electricity of it all was just superb. After that point, I don't remember considering it being hard, or being out of breath. I just remember running. One foot in front of the other, around the course.

For the first time ever, I was running with a huge group of other runners, all heading towards the same goal. I was surrounded by people panting, ploughing and plodding. And it wasn't just super-fit runners either, there were people of all ages, all fitness levels. It was so much fun and I was carried along by the atmosphere, proudly wearing my orange South London top, cheering on our team-mates and exchanging banter with the North Londoners in green.

The North vs South competition gave the whole race a bit of an edge because we all had a purpose. We weren't just running for ourselves, for our own time, we were running for a team and that team was out there, all around us. It was the first time I'd experienced the running community like that. The immediate bond, the cheering each other on, the drive to succeed. Obviously, no PBs were achieved that day – in fact, I couldn't even tell you what time I did. But I do remember crossing the finish line, completely exhausted but absolutely elated.

I did it. I survived! And it was actually a lot of fun.

After that, I was pretty much hooked.

When it comes to races, the support you get from your fellow runners, the crowds that come out to watch and the volunteers that make sure these races can happen are just phenomenal.

UNITED BY A CAUSE

When you do run or attend a race, you will see plenty of people running for charities and causes. Races and fundraising just go together naturally; thousands of people challenge themselves to raise money and awareness for a cause close to their hearts, or maybe just in memory of a loved one.

Whether it's a Race for Life 5K, an obstacle race, a marathon or more, you'll see droves of people in their T-shirts, a rainbow of colours, logos and slogans, punctuated by photos of lost loved ones and those still fighting. Those runners, earning money for those charities, are what keep many of those organisations alive and enable them to continue their brilliant work. It's inspirational and so emotional to watch. The causes you see represented on Race Days can be so diverse, but the drive behind them all is unifying.

The runners we see representing these charities might be strangers, but if we've been affected by these causes directly ourselves or know someone else who has been, we immediately have something in common that is beyond even running. And it motivates people to support you in all sorts of different ways – just take 'Marathon Man' Gary McKee as an example. A fundraiser for Macmillan Cancer Support for almost twenty years, in memory of his dad, who was a cancer survivor, in 2021 he ran 110 marathons in 110 days to celebrate the charity's 110th birthday.

In 2022, Gary went even bigger and decided to run 365 marathons in 365 days. That's right, he ran a marathon EVERY SINGLE DAY for a whole year and raised £1 million for charity. Speaking on *RunPod* as his epic challenge was drawing to a close, he told me about the amazing support he had received in his challenge, with people turning up at his house each day to join on all or part of each of his daily marathons.

'I always think that whatever you're going through, compare that to the people you're raising funds for. Then you can say your day's not as bad as you thought it was,' he said. 'I still get excited wondering who's going to be outside in the morning, because there isn't many days that I've ran alone.'

When he came on the show, 139 people had already completed a full marathon with him.

'For a lot of them it's the first time they've run a marathon so to share that experience is a wonderful warming feeling,' he said. 'Some people leave my house with tears in their eyes, thinking that they would never ever do a marathon, and they just went and smashed one out.'

Something about running for a cause just pushes you on harder and helps you achieve things you didn't think would be possible. I know this from running the marathon for Children's Trust, Cancer Research UK and CLIC Sergeant over the years. You're spurred on to succeed by the people who have put their faith in you, sponsored you and come out, on a day off, to support you. And when it gets hard, the experience of the people you're running for helps you to dig that little bit deeper.

As Gary said: 'I always say that no matter what the rain is like and how hard we're getting hit by it, someone is going to walk out of a cancer ward and they're going to ring the bell to signify that their treatment is over. If they go outside and it's raining, they're going to stand in it, they might even do a little dance and they're going to think it's the nicest rain they've ever felt on their face. I always say to people, "We're running in somebody else's rain."'

Hearing people's stories about why they run, and who they are running for, is so amazing and they break me every time. The running community gets it and whatever the reason you're out running, they will be around you on the course and in the crowds, willing one another to succeed.

Dr Rangan Chatterjee put this feeling of togetherness so beautifully when we chatted about his own London Marathon experience on *RunPod* (see also page 184). He said: 'It wasn't necessarily just the running. What I saw on the day of the London Marathon was people coming together, people supporting each other, lifting other people up. You saw people calling out to people who they literally have never met in their lives and there was this feeling of goodwill, they just wanted people to succeed. And I thought at the end of the day, this is who we are when you leave humans to be humans, interacting with each other in real life. It just really restored my faith in humanity. I know that's pretty deep, but that's honestly my learnings of that day – people want the best in each other.'

That support is what makes you feel a little bit special for that little (or long) period of time that you're running, whether you're doing it for a charity or just to challenge yourself. It's an incredible experience for anyone, as my *RunPod* guest, the Mayor of London, Sadiq Khan, also agreed when we chatted in 2023.

SADIQ'S STORY

A keen runner himself, in addition to having the job of running London, Sadiq got into the sport when he signed up for the London Marathon in 2014. Prior to that he hadn't ran further than seven kilometres, so he wasn't sure he'd be able to do it. Thankfully, the running community lent him a helping hand; encouraged by knowing that people had sponsored him to run and lifted on the day by the crowds and fellow runners, he did it and raised more than £20K for charity.

'I think once you get the bug, once you can run a decent distance, you fall in love – and I fell in love,' he said. 'I've had friends who have done marathons, and half mara-thons and 10Ks, and they say the reason why they did it is because people sponsored them and you feel that responsibility for that – but also because they told people.

'At the London Marathon I probably personally ran twenty-two miles, but the last four-and-a-bit was the crowds. You speak to anybody who has run marathons around the world, they all say London's the best because the crowd sustains you,' he recalled. 'You have your name at the back of your T-shirt and your front, so people cheer you on. First few times you think, *people know who I am*, then you realise … But it's great because of the camarade-rie, that sense of community.

'There are really fit runners going past, going, "Go on, Sadiq" and tapping you on the back, and the last few miles, I kid you not, I must have eaten about 3kg of jelly-beans, because everyone is giving you jellybeans, which you need the sugar to sustain yourself. You also have mates who are running the marathon, who you didn't real-ise were running. My mate Ben was running the marathon and I heard this northern twang "C'mon, Sadiq."

'I thought it could be anybody, right?' he said. 'For a good half a mile he ran with me – even though he's much fitter than me – just to make sure I was going and then I got a second wind and said, "You go" – that sense of commu-nity is hard to explain.'

It's not just the fellow runners that make the London

Marathon special either, it's the spectators and the causes that it supports.

'I've in the past come and cheered on friends that I've known are running,' he said. 'But there's lots of people there who are strangers, they just come along because they may be involved in a charity. People don't realise this but literally tens of millions of pounds are raised in the London Marathon for a variety of charities.

'It's a wonderful day – if you haven't been, it's just a lovely day out. Sometimes the crowds are five-, six-deep, and the diversity of ages, ethnicities, of background,' he added. 'But actually, when I was training for the Marathon and since, you do a half marathon or a 10K, there's a great runners' community there as well and it's really lovely.'

9

PUSHING PAST
YOUR LIMITS

I kid you not, the night before any marathon, I have the exact same dream: I win it. Yup, the whole thing. It goes something like this …

I'd trained as normal and really felt strong as we approached Race Day, then the night before, I slept well and woke up, ready to run and wonder if maybe today I might surprise everyone and put in a good performance. As always, I'm a bundle of nerves, but something happens to me and I just don't burn out or hit the wall – in fact, I simply run gazelle-like, smiling and enjoying every minute.

As I make my way round the course, I hear the crowd cheering, which lifts me even more and then it dawns on me that there aren't any other runners ahead of me. In fact, I'm ahead of the pack. I realise I'm actually just gliding round this marathon course. Yes, I'm feeling a tad tired, but I absolutely can't slow down now. I get to Buckingham Palace and there are only a few hundred yards to go. I pick up my pace, glance around and to my surprise, there is no one else even near me.

I'm living the moment I have always dreamed of. I'm winning the whole thing – out of almost 50,000 people! I burst into a sprint and propel myself across the finish line, arms held high … As people start to run towards me, I realise that I've done it.

I've won the London Marathon!

I had been hoping to get sub-four, completing the race in under four hours, but I'd run even better than expected and finished in just over two hours. It's a miracle and the crowds around me look as surprised as I am.

'I didn't even know I had it in me,' I say.

And that's usually when I wake up.

Now, even though I know it's impossible, for me at least, to win the London Marathon – any marathon, in fact – it's always so vivid that I actually start thinking: *Could I…?* I'm sure I'm not the only person who has this dream of winning the marathon, or any race, quite frankly. We all wonder what it would feel like to achieve the ultimate success, whatever that might look like to you.

Having dreams and goals help us to push ourselves and as a runner, your main competition is almost always yourself. From the moment you start out, you're always trying to get that bit further on your regular route, to run without stopping or just go a tiny bit faster. Then you start aiming for a greater distance, a new PB, maybe even taking on a race … It's exciting, but pushing yourself outside of your comfort zone can be daunting too, like you're standing at the bottom of a mountain wondering how on earth you're going to get to the top. So, how do you prepare yourself to push past your own limits?

WHAT MAKES A CHALLENGE?

Now, winning the London Marathon is just my crazy dream, and while others may share it, it's important to remember that a challenge looks different to everybody. What counts as a challenge can even change for us as individuals as we go through life and experience things like changing jobs, injury, pregnancy and parenthood and your body changing as you age.

Over the years I have run lots of 10Ks and half marathons. While I rarely find them easy, they *are* within my comfort zone. I have also run eight full marathons and prior to having Ella, when I was at my fittest, as I mentioned earlier I was aiming for a 3 hours 15 marathon – a significant challenge for me.

I haven't just got progressively better with every race I've done. Big changes in my life have meant that my capabilities and fitness levels are different now and injuries have meant my goals have had to change. For example, in April 2023, after being injured for months with my glute injury and a frustrating ankle sprain, I did a half marathon for the first time in ages. My goodness, was I excited to race again, but I wasn't able to just pick up where I left off before my injury.

Usually in a half marathon I'd go hell for leather from the start and by the second half would be burnt out but still pushing it, eyeing a new PB. But this time I couldn't do that. Dealing with injury meant that I had to embrace a huge change in mentality and accept that my limits were different. If I didn't change my mindset, I knew I risked aggravating my injury again and ending up with many more months without running.

I had to forget about times, go slow and take care. Just completing the race would be an achievement but it was one that I knew was within my capability. So, I decided to add a slightly crazy element to my plan. I decided to stick to going really slowly through the half marathon, but when I crossed the finish line, I was going to carry on and run the seven miles home afterwards – not far off marathon distance. And do you know what? I did it. I ran easy and still managed to go twenty-five minutes quicker than my training times – my first win of the day. But the icing on the cake was crossing the finish line and realising I could still go on. Through not being able to run, I had realised what a privilege it was and I was taking advantage of every moment. I genuinely wasn't competing with anyone. Instead, I paced myself and was looking around, smiling and taking it all in – I can't tell you just how much I loved that race.

Whenever I'm faced with a big challenge, I always remember something brilliant that running legend and two-times Olympic and Commonwealth gold medallist, Col. Dame Kelly Holmes, MBE, said: 'I believe that things in life are possible, if first you believe they are.' Some people might churn out five or six marathons a year but have an ultramarathon (anything over 26.2 miles) or a race in more challenging conditions, like a desert or the arctic, in their sights. Others again may be working towards a non-stop 10K, a faster 5K or simply just taking part in their first race. None of these challenges is greater or less than the other. We're all at different points in our journey and whatever challenge we choose to take on will push us out of our own comfort zones and past our current limits – they will always feel insurmountable at first. But whether it's going from 5 to 10K, 20 to 40K, or marathon to ultramarathon, it is possible: we *are* capable, we just have to believe it.

SETTING BIG GOALS

There are a couple of times in the year that I enjoy setting running goals. First of all, I think it's quite nice when everyone is making New Year resolutions to spend less, eat fewer crisps, give up alcohol – the type that most of us fail miserably at by 3 January – to make a resolution to *do* something (rather than *not* do something).

You might say you're going to do a parkrun once a month for a whole year or run the whole of a race you once did in a relay on your own. You could take on RED January, which encourages people to 'move every day' throughout the month, or some of you might even be really brave and decide to sign up for an ultramarathon, which by the way, a lot of people say is even more enjoyable than doing a marathon (I haven't done one myself, but I do plan to go down that path at some point – I'm just not there quite yet!). I feel like I get so much more out of these kinds of goals than the ones focused on deprivation – they're much more fun!

The other time I get the urge to set a new challenge is what I consider to be 'Runners' New Year' – the day after the London Marathon. It's no surprise that the ballot for the following year's race opens on the weekend of the event. The excitement, the emotion, the atmosphere – the organisers know *exactly* how it all affects people. Whether you ran it yourself and are still riding your runner's high, or you watched in the crowd or at home, got inspired and started thinking, *I could do that* …, it just gets you thinking about what might be possible, if you put your mind to it.

I like to have a challenge or race to focus on in the spring, and another one in autumn, so I'll be training January to April before taking the summer off (no one wants to be training eighteen-milers on their holidays!) and start training again in August for a race in October. Of course, there are races all year round and you can set your goals at any time, using the goal-setting techniques I shared in Chapter 2 (see also page 37). Just make sure that whatever goal you do set, it's 'SMART' and something you really want to do, especially if it requires significant training. You see, if your heart's not in it, you will set yourself up for failure at worst, or an unpleasant experience at best – and no one wants either of those things!

FIND YOUR PROCESS

Once you've decided on your goal, you have to break it down and work out how you're going to get there. Now, we will all have a slightly different process when we prepare for a challenge, but the fundamentals are usually the same. The best way I can illustrate this is sharing how I prepare for my biggest and favourite challenge – running the London Marathon.

Despite the fact that I have run eight and trained for twelve of them, a marathon is still a really big deal. For me it's a once-a-year thing and my chance to really push and see what I can achieve. It's certainly not something I do multiple times a year – or on a daily basis, like 'marathon man' Gary McKee (see also page 210), nor is it something I can just turn up and 'do' – I need to train, focus and really build up to it.

The London Marathon was actually the second race that I ever ran. I was asked by The Children's Trust, the UK's leading charity helping children with brain injury, to run it on their behalf and I agreed immediately. I'd loved the whole race experience at the North vs South 10K and already found watching the London Marathon so inspiring, so why not?

But I had no idea what I was getting into.

The time goal that I set myself was plucked out of thin air. I'd heard lots of people say they had a 'sub-four' marathon, so I decided that I would try and do the race in under four hours. So, I downloaded the training plan for a three-hour forty-five-minute marathon from the marathon website and off I went.

CONSIDER YOUR SCHEDULE

Now, had I known more about what training for a marathon involved, I might have given the challenge a lot more consideration. I certainly do nowadays. So many people sign up and think, *I can fit that in around my two jobs, three children and social life*, without fully understanding the reality of the timescales involved and the training required for a race.

Before you sign up to any race or challenge, make sure you check out what training is required for the level that you are currently at and how long before the race you need to start – just to make sure it's realistic. When it comes to a marathon, you really have to consider whether you have the time and energy to commit. Your heart and mind must both be in it, your body has to be able to do it and you must look after yourself along the way to avoid injury or long-term damage. So, whatever you do, don't try to squeeze three months of training into one month or take on a challenge when you're overloaded with work or family commitments. Instead, maybe put it off until next year, or look for another race that offers the same challenge but gives you an appropriate timescale to train.

Self-belief is vital and yes, anyone can do a marathon – or really whatever race it is that you might have signed up for. But to make sure you complete it and, most importantly, *enjoy* it, you have to make sure you've done all the right things. To do that, you'll need time and a training plan.

GET A TRAINING PLAN

The experience of taking on a challenge like a marathon isn't just Race Day. And it's not just getting the medal and bragging about it. The experience starts the minute you sign up and takes in everything running up to the race – people often forget this.

This is why having a training plan is a vital part of the experience. It's the blueprint for your whole race experience. Now, I know many people who haven't trained for the marathon, who have just turned up and tried to wing it. From what I've witnessed, all that happens in these cases is that you do it, you're in pain and you hate it. You'll be tired and broken afterwards, maybe even injured, and you'll take ages to recover. You won't cross the finish line cheering and delighted, you'll just be put off running for life when it really didn't have to be that way.

To get the most out of the race, you have to really put a circle around Race Day in the diary and work towards it, count down and get excited by the process as much as the outcome.

I can't state this strongly enough. Do not ruin your own marathon experience: GET A TRAINING PLAN!

Now, there are a gazillion marathon training programmes out there and one of them is right for you – but which one? That is the killer question. Everyone has different needs, our schedules all vary so we don't all have the same availability, so there really is no one-size-fits-all and everything you'll find out there is largely generic.

If you want a bespoke training plan that is tailored to you and your specific goal, you will need to work with a running coach, who will develop a training plan for you. But, if you need something to simply get you to the finish line, or an idea of the kind of thing you should be trying to tick off in the time leading up to Race Day, I have written an example of a marathon training programme that I have followed myself, which you can find on page 265.

Also, when it comes to training plans, I don't know many people who stick to them religiously. See your plan as a guide not an instruction manual. It is not set in stone, you can be flexible with it – to fit it all in, you will need to be sometimes because life can get in the way. If you miss a run, don't stress. If you get a cold, then relax and recover, don't fret. Energy levels change, you might ache or feel tired, so just be kind to yourself. If at all you feel yourself wearing out, or a little niggle, back off even just for a day. Never be scared of a bonus rest day – you have plenty of time to work up to Race Day!

TELL PEOPLE WHAT YOU'RE DOING

You might find that the first few weeks of marathon training feel easy, but *do not* get cocky, it'll toughen up before you know it. After all, it's meant to be hard. If it was easy, wouldn't everyone do it? If it was easy, why would anyone sponsor you, or come out to cheer you on?

Training is intense and you'll need the people in your life to know that, for a period of time, it is going to be your focus. This means that perhaps you might not be out as much, or you'll be using your weekends for long training runs rather than your usual activities.

Now, remember that most people have no idea what's involved in training for a marathon (even less so an ultra or other less common running challenge), so tell them! Stick your weekly training plan on the fridge as a reminder for you and anyone else what your training commitments are. If your friends, colleagues and family fully understand what you're doing, they'll be there to cheer you on, keep you on track and be far less likely to accidentally derail you with plans that just don't fit in.

Beyond your close family and friends, sharing your goal publicly, on social media or in an online running community for example, is also a great way to get even more accountability and keep yourself on track with training. If you're fundraising too, sharing your training journey might also help generate donations!

GET STUCK IN

Once you have your goal, your training plan and your people supporting you, all that's left to do is get stuck into your training. When I'm training for a marathon, I like to stick to a sixteen-week training programme, like my marathon plan on page 265.

Now, the great thing about this is if you're aiming to run the London, Brighton or Manchester Marathons, they all take place in April, so your sixteen weeks usually starts on the first day of January. It's likely to be cold, dark and a bit boring. Most of us are trying to be healthy at the start of a new year and suddenly having a training programme means that the month no longer drags, it gives you some focus – it really is the perfect time to get stuck into a challenge. But what does marathon training actually look like?

My marathon plan is based on running four times a week because that's what I like to do. If you're following it though, the fourth run can be optional, so if life gets in the way, that's the one you can miss guilt-free.

Each week you need a long run – this is key, as it's training your body to run a long way. The marathon is 26.2 miles, so you need to get some 'miles in the legs', so you know what that feels like. These long runs should be done at an easy pace and it's absolutely not a failure if you do some walking – getting the miles in is what matters! You also need a faster run each week – a run with the pace that you would love to pull out of the bag on marathon day. You need to get used to how that feels, or even just work out what that pace actually is. However, if you don't have a marathon pace, don't panic, simply run at a comfortable pace. It's more important to get the runs in the bag.

Speedwork (tempo runs) and hill sprints will also help to build up endurance and strength in the legs.

Your running days should be spread out, definitely not all back-to-back. You should aim for a day off between, but if you do have some days that you run back-to-back, go for an easy run, combined with a tempo or hill session. Every week in a marathon training programme you add a little bit more to the 'long run', then every few weeks, it drops back a bit to give you an easy week before ramping it up again – this means that you're always getting a breather.

Out of your sixteen weeks, there will be thirteen weeks of ramping up and three weeks of tapering – the bit at the end when you are just waiting for Race Day. This bit is important. Don't save your longest training run for the week before the marathon, the taper period is designed to help you get in optimum condition. As well as scheduling your runs and getting the correct mix to ensure you're fully prepared, remember that you also need to supplement your running with other training too.

DO THE EXTRA WORK (AND REST)

While working towards your marathon or other running goal, you should try to fit in some training that is *not* running where you can, maybe cross-training, a strength and conditioning session using weights in the gym, or even cycling – something that will complement your running work. If you choose to do strength training, you don't even have to go to a gym, you can try the bodyweight exercises I recommended in Chapter 5 (see also pages 125–31). So many muscles are weak from only running that working on your core, upper body, glutes, upper legs and hips will help you in the mission to stay strong and avoid injury.

Similarly, make sure you make time for recovery, factoring in rest days and post-run ice baths. I also tend to book myself a sports massage every few weeks during marathon training to loosen up tight areas and identify any potential niggles that could turn into injuries. I tend to have my last one a few days before the race and I also book one for a few days after as part of my post-race recovery.

'MARANOIA' AND OTHER DOUBTS

The closer Race Day gets, the more doubts may start to set in. You might question what you were thinking when you signed up and wondering if you're in over your head.

When Col. Dame Kelly Holmes, MBE, joined me on *RunPod* (see also page 219), she talked about this on the journey of trying to achieve a goal. She highlighted how moments of self-doubt and thinking that you're 'not good enough' are natural and how we should look back on how far we have come to give us the confidence to overcome these doubts.

'What people don't do is look back on what they came from. They only think of where they have not yet got to,' she observed. 'I think people have to look back at where they started and believe in themselves that they can continue the journey and that they will get better.'

So, when the doubts start to creep in, take a moment to think back to where your journey started; consider the first time you went for a run. If you'd told yourself on that day, that one day you'd have run an eighteen-mile training run, would you have believed them? Probably not. But look, you've done it! You've already achieved more than you once thought you were capable of, so why won't you do it again?

After three weeks of tapering in a marathon plan, you should be like a coiled spring ready to go when the starting gun is fired. But this is also when 'maranoia' can arise – paranoia about the marathon (an experience I'm sure isn't exclusive just to marathoners and likely affects anyone who has been training for a big challenge).

You will think you're injured, you're eating too much, you're not eating enough, you're dehydrated, you're going to have a horrible race and get a terrible time – just about every possible issue goes through your mind. By this point you have invested four months of your life in training, so once again, the fear that it might all end up being for nothing is completely natural. But don't let it tarnish your experience, instead try these things:

* Focus on the process – Enjoy achieving the smaller goals that you've mapped out – the weekly runs in your plan and other training sessions – rather than obsessing about the final outcome. If you do those, you'll be ready for the big day!

* Look after yourself, body and mind – Eat well, sleep plenty, hydrate and prioritise recovery. Do the things that support your mental health too, like getting out for a walk, meditating or practising mindfulness.

* Talk to people – You know the people that you told about your big challenge at the start, the online community you shared it with? They are your support network, so talk to them about your worries. Non-running friends and family will be able to lend a sympathetic ear, while fellow runners will likely be able to provide support and advice.

* Make a game plan for the day – Particularly if it's your first marathon, you might be anxious about the practicalities of the day: what you're going to eat and when, how you're getting to the start line, what you're going to wear. If you map it all out in advance, you'll find you feel a whole lot more relaxed.

THE FINAL COUNTDOWN ...

As the marathon gets closer, as well as starting to think about the logistics of the day, there are a few other things to turn your attention to. One is what you are eating and drinking.

I don't have a particular nutrition plan, but in the month before the marathon, I do try to eat as healthy and balanced a diet as possible, cutting out any rubbish so my body is properly fuelled. I still go out, see friends and socialise normally, but when I'm focused on my training, I eat better and I also tend not to drink alcohol for the month before the race.

Now, there's no hard and fast rule on when – or indeed if – you should stop drinking alcohol before a race, although I don't think anyone would recommend a marathon with a hangover! It really is down to the individual, but there's a broad recommendation that you shouldn't drink forty-eight hours before a race because your glycogen storage (where you're going to be getting your energy from) is reduced the day after drinking.

Hydration ahead of the race is also important and trying to do that on the morning of the race is a bit like last-minute cramming for an exam: it's not all going to stay in. I make sure that I drink plenty of water in the week running up to the race and I carry a big bottle with me to the marathon start line and sip from it continuously until the race is ready to begin.

Finally, if you've got shiny, fancy new kit for Race Day, make sure you wear it a few times on your training runs to make sure it's comfortable and doesn't chafe – that's definitely not something you want to discover on the day itself!

MARATHON EVE: PASTA PARTY

Looking through the magazine and training plan that I'd downloaded for my first marathon, I remember spotting: 'Carb loading – pasta party' as an event. Intrigued, I learnt that the night before the race, lots of participants go to the Marathon Expo (where you go to get your number and event pack in the days leading up to the race) to eat loads of pasta and socialise.

Now, I had already collected my pack, so I wasn't planning on going back to the expo, but I was utterly convinced that carb-loading on pasta was an absolute essential. It was about six o'clock when I started cooking a vat of pasta with tomato sauce.

'This is what everyone does,' I told James as I pulled out our biggest salad bowl and poured the pasta in. 'I have to carb-load.'

So I ate an *entire* salad bowl of pasta with tomato sauce. It was an enormous portion, and even when I was full up, I kept on going until I'd finished it all. I honestly believed it was what I had to do.

Now, I've since learnt that eating a salad bowl full of pasta is *not* an essential part of night-before marathon prep. In fact, it's a bit of a myth and just makes you need to stop at a portable loo more on the way round. Food-wise, I've found it's more than enough to just add some extra carbs to your meals and make sure you're having a portion of protein with each meal in the days leading up to the race. Simple as that. Eliud Kipchoge, the GOAT of marathons (see also page 148), has some rice before his races, but not a salad bowl-size portion. Now, if you *want* your pasta party, go for it. I just want you to know that although it might be fun, it's not the essential that some people might have you believe.

Food sorted, all that's left to do the night before is to get your time-tracking chip attached to your trainers, your number pinned to your shirt (you don't want to be messing around with these jobs in the morning) and lay out all your kit, clothes and trainers, ready for the big day. At this point, you've done all you can so just watch some TV to help you relax, get a good night's sleep and enjoy those sweet dreams of crossing the finish line!

RACE DAY

If you've never done a marathon before – and actually, even if you have – it's super nerve-wracking, but so exciting too. In fact, the London Marathon is my favourite day of the whole year.

I get up in the morning, buzzing and full of nerves – this is the runner's equivalent of a child on Christmas morning. Then I put my kit on, get all my gels in my running belt. I have a cup of tea, water and a dry bagel – which I know is so boring, but it's become my traditional pre-marathon breakfast. Now, it's time to head to the race start at Greenwich in Southeast London. As you make your way across London, you start seeing runners everywhere. Every train going to that part of town is filled with runners from around the country and around the world, coming from all parts of the city where they live or have been staying.

Eventually everyone gets on the train to Greenwich – you might call it the 'Lycra train' – basically a one-way trip to the start line packed with anxious and excited marathoners, and barely a non-runner in sight! At first no one speaks, but then inevitably, someone will ask: 'So, have you done this before?' And that's it. That's all it takes to set the entire train off. The questions start off, identifying who's a newbie and who's done a marathon before: '*First marathon?*', '*No, fifth, all London*', '*It's my first!*'. Then it slides into training: *When did you start? How much have you done? Do you think you're ready?* Let me tell you, no one ever says: '*Yeah, I'm fully trained. I had a great night's sleep and I'm absolutely ready to take on this race.*' Instead, all you hear is, *I'm so nervous. I feel sick. I need the toilet.*

Chatter then slips into practicalities: *Does anyone have any water? Are there toilets en route to the start? Are you using gels?* This can turn into blind panic in some: *I've forgotten my gels! Does anyone have any spares?* It's just all runners, all nervous, all panicking, all stressing about the same race. The whole train becomes a vibrating hive of collective nerves and angst, but in a strange way it's lovely, because everyone is there looking out for one another.

Water is being passed around, gels are shared, veterans tell first-timers what they're about to experience – everyone is trying to put one another at ease. No matter how many times I do it, I'm always nervous on Race Day but the excitement and feeling of being part of something helps me through it. By the time you come out of the station and you reach the race start, I promise you, you'll be ready and raring to go!

YOUR LAP OF HONOUR

Even though when you're on the 'Lycra train' to the start line, you're maybe an hour or so away from beginning your marathon experience, you can't help but ask those who've done it before what *exactly* is about to happen. The best way to describe it is that Race Day is your lap of honour. The training is the hard work and you've done all that. Now, this is your moment to just get out there and enjoy it.

The chatter from the train continues as you gather: *How are you feeling? What time are you hoping for? Oh, I love your trainers!* People are laughing, getting their watches ready, trying to find their GPS and it's all fun and exciting. Then there's a second when the mood switches. Watch any start line and the same thing happens. It could be your local parkrun or the New York Marathon. As people get towards the start, it goes from smiley to serious as they enter 'running focus' mode. As you cross the start line there's a cacophony of beeps as watches go on and you can just see in everyone's expressions that they're thinking, *Right, we're off. Let's do this.*

You start running and inside your mind is screaming, *I'm in a race, I'm in a race, I'm in a race. Oh, my goodness, I'm in a race!*

It's game face, but for all of about ten seconds.

After that, you settle into it and realise it's just a run, only with loads of other people who love running too. And it's likely to be the most enjoyable run you've ever done because there's no waiting at traffic lights, no stopping at the zebra crossing, no weaving around bicycles and other obstacles you usually come across. The roads are empty except for you and thousands of other runners. There's water on demand, energy gels being handed out, toilets en route and even showers to run through.

Everything is geared towards you – the runner. It's lovely!

On top of that, you get to experience the crowds cheering you on too. Thousands of people have come out to watch YOU and your fellow runners in awe. They're there to be inspired, support you and celebrate you doing something remarkable with your day, whether that's raising money for charity or just pushing yourself to do something you've never done before.

There'll be parts of the route where there are no crowds, when you'll just be surrounded by runners and all you hear is panting – that's the perfect time to take a quiet moment to watch other people, acknowledge yourself as a runner and really take in the amazing thing that you're doing. On the way round you might see friends, colleagues, people you spoke to on the train, or someone you saw at your local tube station hours earlier as you headed to join the Lycra-clad pilgrimage to Greenwich, running alongside you. You'll smile and wave and encourage one another to keep on going.

The endorphins will well and truly be pumping, but there is truly no moment in any race like the one when you cross the finish line. If you've got friends and family cheering you on, this is where they'll be screaming for you. It might be hugely emotional because it's something that you never thought possible. You might look back to where you were a year ago and think, *Look how far I've come. I never thought that I'd sign up for a race, let alone head*

238

towards a finish line. But here you are. Your heart will be pounding, your legs will feel like jelly, but you'll want to dig in and finish strong. You'll also suddenly think, *How am I going to finish?* – because everyone wants a great finish-line photo to look back on!

Now, as I've learnt, if you don't commit to your training, what you end up with is a photo of you slumped forward and projectile vomiting across the line – not the greatest look! Nowadays, I recommend training properly and aiming for a sprint finish for the last 100 metres or so. I'll look at my watch, look at the finish line and decide what time I'm going to make it there by. Even if the 'sprint' I muster is little more than a slow shuffle, it makes me feel like I've given it my all, right up to the last second. And as you cross the finish line and finally get your medal – that exciting bit of bling you've been after for so long – that's when it will really kick in: the adrenaline, the joy, the elation, the ultimate runner's high.

Your lap of honour is complete – you did it!

There are so, so many great reasons to enter a race, or to set yourself a challenge, not least having a great story to tell when you go into work the next day. But for me, the greatest reason of all is just to push yourself outside of your comfort zone, defy any limits you think you have and find out what you're really capable of, all while having a wonderful time.

After all, anything is possible if first you believe it is.

MARK'S STORY

Now, if you ever start to think that you might not be capable of achieving a goal you've set for yourself, or that you've achieved all you are capable of, I urge you to listen to my *RunPod* episode from November 2022 with the incredible Mark Ormrod, MBE, a former Royal Marine, Invictus Games athlete, motivational speaker – and triple amputee.

If anyone proves that you can push yourself past any limits, it's Mark. On Christmas Eve 2008, at the age of twenty-four, while on routine foot patrol, he triggered an improvised explosive device (IED) that resulted in injuries, leading to him having one arm and both legs above the knee amputated. But rather than be defeated by his injuries, Mark focused his mindset on overcoming them.

'It was difficult. I was twenty-four years old. A week before, I'd been 6ft 2in, weighed 16 stone and was physically approaching my peak,' he told me. 'I was a Royal Marines Commando; I had the best job in the world and that had all been taken away from me in a heartbeat. I'd lost my career, my identity, everything that I prided myself on was gone.

'A doctor told me that I had zero chance of ever walking again, because he had never met anyone missing one leg above the knee that had any success using prosthetics because they were too painful, too difficult to use, and they took too much energy that no one had ever achieved it,' he said. 'And that was somebody missing just one leg.'

Six days later, Mark had another visitor, a man who also had two missing legs, but had learnt to walk on prosthetics. Inspired by his story and what he had achieved, Mark decided not to give up.

'I started thinking, *I'm still a Royal Marine, I'm just not going to wear a uniform anymore. I still have the standards, the values, the ethos within me and that's what I'm going to carry forward into my rehab and then into my life*,' he said. 'And it was a complete mindset shift for me – it motivated me, it fired me up and it gave me a bigger purpose than just myself.'

Following twelve months of rehab, Mark started searching for support. He found a triple amputee like himself who ran Dream Team Prosthetics and arranged to go to America to be trained by them for three weeks. As well as teaching him to run and swim in his new prosthetics, the team even made him enter the Endeavour Games – a mini version of the Invictus Games – where he had to compete using his newly-learnt skills and techniques.

'I'll be honest with you, I never liked running. But I think now would be different, if I was able-bodied now, because I understand a lot more about technique,' he said. 'Initially [when learning to run on blades], I had to run into cars and brick walls to stop, because the blade almost acts like a spring – it kind of springs you forward once you get the technique right. But once you get up a head of steam, I found it very difficult to stop.

'Eventually, you learn your body position, you lean back a little bit, drop your bum a bit to act as a brake, but the energy expenditure is horrendous. For a double above-knee amputee, running is probably 600 to 800 per cent more intensive than an able-bodied person because you drive everything from your glutes, your hips and your lower back,' he continued. 'You don't have calves, your quads don't work, your hamstrings don't work, you don't have knees or ankles or toes or anything to drive with, you have just got to do it all from what you've got left. Even having an arm missing – I've got a little bit left of the other one, but it's not enough to provide that swing and that momentum to drive you forwards – you kind of have to work out how to use the leg to its most efficient.

'They pushed me to my limits and beyond it and taught me how to live,' he added. 'I came back from America and I wanted to start challenging myself. I'd been heavily supported by military charities, so I wanted to figure some challenges out and combine it with fundraising and try and give back a little bit and say thank you to these organisations that had supported me and my family.'

In 2010 Mark ran with friends from New York to LA – 3,500 miles across America, cycled from Mark's hometown of Plymouth anticlockwise around the UK, 3,200 miles, and did skydiving, bungee jumping and a few other 'little' things, taking him up to 2016, when he was sat in his home office writing his goals for the following year.

'I'd never done any sport competitively since I'd been injured. I had seen friends of mine at the Invictus Games. It was two years old at this point and 2017, Christmas Eve, was going to be my ten-year anniversary,' he said. 'So, I thought, that's going to be a good way to celebrate ten years of life post-injury.

'I didn't know if I was capable of learning these sports and then training in them and learning the rules and the strategies and the technique,' he said. 'But I just thought I'd give it a shot and see what happens. I applied and I was very fortunate that I got in the team. And then I was like, OK, cool. Now I have to learn how to row, how to swim, how to handcycle, how to do shot put and discus and all these things.'

Training at home during the week and travelling to Invictus Games camps around the UK at the weekend, Mark figured out what worked for him and what didn't before he went and competed. In 2017 he won two silver medals in rowing and two bronze in the pool, and when he returned in 2018, he added four golds and a silver to his medal haul. When I asked him why he does what he does, his answer has stuck with me: 'I can, so I should.'

'I do it first of all because I can. And I am grateful for the fact that I can. I have friends who are more severely injured than myself who would love to be able to go out there and run and swim, but unfortunately their situation means that they can't, so I don't take that for granted. I love the fact that I can do this and I think that if I can, I should,' he said. 'And I enjoy it – being physically active has a huge impact on my mental health, it always keeps me strong, keeps me focused, keeps me moving forward. If I was a doctor, this is what I would prescribe: Any form of physical activity that you're passionate about, do it more often.'

If we can, we should – so what challenge are you going to set for yourself?

TEST YOUR LIMITS: ALTERNATIVE RACES

Now, as you might have noticed, I think marathons are incredible, but I know that they're not everyone's cup of tea. Also, you shouldn't restrict yourself when it comes to running goals. Outside of traditional distances and formats, there's a whole lot to choose from. You might want something that involves more teamwork, something more playful and a bit silly, or something that is much, much more challenging. Whatever it is that you're looking for, why not consider some of these alternative challenges from around the world?

Marathon du Médoc

The Marathon du Médoc is a marathon race unlike any other. Held every year in September through the vineyards of the Médoc in the Gironde, north of Bordeaux. It's basically a gastro marathon, where you drink wine provided by the vineyards you pass through as you go, with ice cream and champagne served over the last few kilometres. One *RunPod* guest, the adventure athlete and journalist, Tobias Mews, actually did this for his wedding, with everyone in fancy dress and the bride and groom acting as pacemakers. It was the majority of his guests' first marathon!

Now, the aim of this race is definitely not about smashing a PB. It's exactly the opposite – in fact, most participants aim for a 'Personal Worst'. The race is nicknamed *'le marathon le plus long du monde'* – the longest marathon in the world – and with 11,000 people drinking their way around twenty vineyards in a six-and-a-half-hour window, that's no real surprise!

Walt Disney World Marathon Weekend

Take on a 5K, 10K, half or full marathon in Walt Disney World. Get dressed up, meet your favourite characters (I even sacrificed an improved time to get my photo with Minnie Mouse!) and explore the park before it opens to the public for the day – a challenge and a truly magical experience.

Run Alton Towers

Disney a bit too far? You can do a 5K, 10K or half marathon at Alton Towers, exploring ten themed areas and spanning over 500 acres before getting to enjoy all the rides!

Whole Earth Man v Horse

An event began in June 1980 following a discussion in the back bar of The Neuadd Arms Hotel, in Llanwrtyd Wells, debating whether a man or a horse would run faster over mountainous terrain. Landlord Gordon Green decided to put it to the test and the Man v Horse race was born. It's exactly as it sounds: men (and women) race a horse across a 22.5-mile course to see who comes out on top. Only four humans have ever beaten the horse but it's possible, so definitely worth a shot!

Obstacle Courses

If you want some variety in your race, an obstacle course might be the ideal challenge for you. There are loads of options, from the family-friendly Cancer Research Pretty Muddy 5K to Tough Mudder's 15K course, which features lots of running between obstacles ranging from a freezing plunge into icy water or scrambling up a giant climbing frame to crawling through muddy pits and swinging on monkey bars (your strength training will come in handy here). Also, check out Spartan Races, inflatable obstacle races, colour runs, light runs, neon runs ... the list is endless!

Dragon's Back Race (Ras Cefn y Ddraig)

A multi-day running race down the 'spine of Wales', covering 380 kilometres of mountains from Conway Castle in North Wales to Cardiff Castle in South Wales. This trail-running experience passes through incredibly challenging terrain as you take in breathtaking scenery and really push yourself to your limits. If you're not quite ready for the full route, the 'Hatchling' option allows you to participate in just part of the race each day.

Race the Train

Race the Train is an annual cross-country running event that takes place in Tywyn, mid-Wales, and attracts runners from all over the world. There's a series of races, including a 'Toddlers Trot' for children up to the age of nine, but the main event sees runners compete to beat a steam train on the preserved Talyllyn Railway over a distance of fourteen miles.

Spartathlon

A historic ultra-distance race in Greece, ideal for experienced runners who also love a bit of history! The Spartathlon revives the footsteps of Pheidippides, an ancient Athenian messenger who, before the Battle of Marathon in 490 BC, was sent to Sparta to get help in the war between the Greeks and the Persians. According to an ancient Greek historian, he arrived in Sparta the day after his departure from Athens – covering 250 kilometres within thirty-six hours. Participants take on the same gruelling challenge, crossing muddy paths, vineyards, olive groves, climb steep hillsides and there is a 1,200-metre ascent and descent of Mount Parthenion, all in the middle of the night. Not for the fainthearted!

Wife Carrying Race

Take on a challenging obstacle course in Dorking, Surrey, set over sand, water and fences – all to be navigated while carrying your partner in a test of communication, stamina and physical strength. Your partner doesn't have to be your legal wife, but they certainly do need to trust you. Oh, and by the way, the winner gets the wife's weight in beer (and bragging rights, of course!). The official Wife Carrying World Championships are held every year in Sonkajärvi, Finland, but there are similar wife carrying events that now take place all over the world, if it sounds like your kind of thing!

The Polar Circle Marathon

Dubbed 'the coolest marathon on earth', the Polar Circle Marathon takes place in Kangerlussuaq, Greenland, across ice and arctic tundra, in one of the most remote corners of the world. A weekend event, you can take on the full marathon on Saturday or half marathon on Sunday – or run both by joining the 'Polar Bear Challenge'!

Marathon des Sables

At the other end of the temperature extreme is 'the toughest footrace on earth'. The Marathon des Sables takes place over six days in the Sahara Desert in Morocco. Running more than 250 kilometres (approximately six full marathons) across sand dunes, rocky jebels (mountains) and white-hot salt plains, carrying what you need to survive on your back, this isn't just a physical challenge, it's a mental challenge too.

CONCLUSION

Running just seems to have a way of finding you and once it does, there's no shaking it off. For months and months before I pulled on my trainers for the first time, there were so many little nudges: noticing joggers in the street and wondering if it was for me, the excitement of seeing the London Marathon on TV and my boss at the time finally talking me into giving it a try. So many of the people I speak to who are already running have a similar story. Once you start considering it, running is suddenly everywhere, until you finally go for it. And when you do, oh my goodness, what a feeling! The burning lungs, the racing heart and that soaring sense of achievement that has you beaming from ear to ear – it's that undeniable runner's high that gets you hooked and keeps you pounding the pavements.

I am eternally grateful to the younger version of myself who dragged herself out of her flat on that bitterly cold

Glasgow day, fashion trainers on and CD Walkman stuffed in bra, and just ran. From that first runner's high I found a lifelong passion, one that has shaped my life in so many ways – the experiences I've had, the friends I've made and even the places I've been – and it continues to bring me so much joy.

If you were needing a final nudge to get out there, or to take on your next challenge, I hope that this book has been it. Running can be the key to a door that opens up a whole world of amazing opportunities and experiences, whether that's exploring new places, meeting new people, challenging yourself physically or giving your mental health a boost by getting headspace and clarity. But if you're still having doubts or you need a reminder about why you do this crazy, brilliant thing called running, here's a few things for you to consider.

RUNNING IS FOR ANYONE AND IT'S NEVER TOO LATE TO START

The greatest thing about running is that almost anyone can run and you can start at any time – all you need is the time and your trainers. People often find themselves being told (or telling themselves) that they're too old to run, or that it's too late to start but that's just not the case. Take my neighbour's dad, for example. After seeing how much his son enjoyed running, he decided to give it a try and started running in his sixties. Now in his late-seventies, he's still running marathons. In the *RunPod* Run Club Facebook group as well, there are so many members who took up running when they were older and can't believe they didn't do it sooner – which brings me to my next point …

YOU'LL NEVER REGRET A RUN

I've said it before, and I'll say it again, you'll never regret going for a run, but you might regret *not* going for one. I have spoken to hundreds of runners and interviewed many for the podcast and when regrets arise, it's usually only in the context of having not done a run; perhaps missing a race or waiting a long time to even try running in the first place. No one really ever talks about wishing they hadn't done a run. Even if it's not a great run, or a particularly enjoyable one, the fact that you've done it means you have achieved something – and that will leave you feeling good and regret-free.

RUNNING CHANGES AS YOU DO

I've been running for almost three decades now and I'm a completely different person to who I was when I first started out. I'm not young, single and child-free anymore, I'm a mum with a busy career, so my ability to train is very different. My fitness levels have changed, I've faced injuries and I've had to reassess my running goals. After I ran my first London Marathon, fifteen years ago, I was so set on getting my next PB, but now I'm more focused on training in a way that means I'll be able to keep running way into the future because I always want to be able to do this thing that I love so much. Fortunately, running can move with you as your life changes. You don't have to give it up just because you're a mum, or because you changed jobs or had an injury, you can adapt how you run, where you run and why you run to suit any stage of your life – so, if you don't want to, you never have to give it up!

YOU'LL ALWAYS HAVE A COMMUNITY

You can be anywhere in the world, anywhere, and if you meet another runner, I guarantee that you'll be able to chat for hours. It's a common bond that seems to transcend all others and I think that's really special. As I said at the very start of this book, from the moment that your trainers hit the pavement on your first run, you're in the gang. And it really is the best gang to be in. You might be crossing paths with a fellow runner on a new route in a new city, sharing your latest run selfie online, or flagging the middle of a pack of runners during a race – wherever it is, the running community will be there to welcome you, celebrate your success, or pick you up and keep you going when it's tough. Being part of such a positive, encouraging and global community is a powerful thing, and if you're a runner, you'll always be connected.

BE YOUR OWN MAIN COMPETITION

While there's plenty of opportunity to be competitive as a runner, you should always be your own main competition. There are so many ways to test your limits in running. Sometimes it's hard not to look at what others are doing and compare your goals and achievements to theirs, but you really don't need to. You don't have to do that marathon just because everyone else is, you can stick to getting a faster 5K, or just running a little bit further without stopping. As the saying goes, comparison is the thief of joy and this is as true of running as it is anywhere else. Don't focus on what other people are doing, challenge yourself to improve on your last run, to achieve things you never thought possible for you, and never let striving for success suck the fun out of a great run.

YOUR RUNNER'S HIGH IS UNIQUE, EMBRACE IT!

We all come from different backgrounds, we run in different ways and for a variety of reasons. We all have varying abilities and goals that are personal to us as individuals, but we are all unified by our love of the freedom and the joy that a good run brings us – that runner's high. But it's important to remember that no two runner's highs are the same. It's not a single feeling that we all experience in the same way, at the same time. It hits us all different ways and it can even change over time. It might be the feeling you get as you realise that you've reached your usual rest point, but have been able to keep on running, the euphoric rush as you stumble across the finish line of a race, or the sensation of running along a glorious seafront, sun on your face and breeze in your hair. Every runner's high you experience is totally unique, completely yours and there to be embraced and enjoyed – every single time.

Getting started really is just the beginning of your running journey. What happens after your first run is entirely up to you and that's the true beauty of this sport. You can run for fun, for fitness, or for the sense of achievement; for the community, for the chance to be out in nature, or just for that feeling of release after a hard day at work … whatever it is that you need from running, it's there for the taking. The road is open and stretching in front of you. So, what are you waiting for? Get out there and find your runner's high!

APPENDIX: TRAINING PROGRAMMES

These training plans are a guideline only and should not replace advice from your healthcare provider. If you are new to regular exercise, or returning after a break, please seek advice from a healthcare professional before starting.

THE *RUNPOD* 5K CHALLENGE

Devised by celebrity trainer and 'Mr PMA' Faisal Abdalla.
In a few weeks' time you're going to run 5K, all in one go. That's right, so get used to it! But first, some advice:

✳ For maximum enjoyment (and lots of encouragement) complete each run while listening to the corresponding *RunPod* episode.

* Spend at least one week on each block, but if you need longer that's fine too.

* Unless otherwise advised, run at a comfortable pace that you can maintain and try not to stop in 'run' segments.

* You can repeat these runs as many times as you like!

* Have a rest day between runs.

* Why not join the *RunPod* Run Club Facebook group and share your journey?

Getting Started (Episode Date: 5 January 2020)

Map the 5K route you're going to run.

Walk it – don't worry about the time, just complete it.

Block One (Episode Date: 12 January 2020)

Repeat this a minimum of three times.

Warm up: Five-minute brisk walk (like you're walking fast to catch a bus, or because it's cold).

Run sixty seconds (maintain that work rate).

Active rest ninety seconds (walk or stand on the spot with light movement).

Repeat x seven.

Run sixty seconds.

Cool down: Walk for five minutes to bring your heart rate down, or try some of Faisal's cool-down exercises on his

PMA Fitness YouTube Channel.

Block Two (Episode Date: 19 January 2020)
Repeat this a minimum of three times.

Warm up: Five-minute brisk walk.
Run one minute thirty seconds.
Walk two minutes.
Repeat x seven.
Run one minute thirty seconds.
Cool down: Walk for five minutes to bring your heart rate down, or try some of Faisal's cool-down exercises on his PMA Fitness YouTube Channel.

Block Three
Run One (Episode Date: 26 January 2020)

Warm up: Five-minute brisk walk.
Run five minutes.
Walk three minutes.
Repeat x two.
Run five minutes.
Cool down: Walk for five minutes to bring your heart rate down, or try some of Faisal's cool-down exercises on his PMA Fitness YouTube Channel.

Run Two (Episode Date: 28 January 2020)

Warm up: Five-minute brisk walk.
Run eight minutes.
Walk five minutes.
Run eight minutes.
Cool down: Walk for five minutes to bring your heart rate down, or try some of Faisal's cool-down exercises on his PMA Fitness YouTube Channel.

Run Three (Episode Date: 30 January 2020)

Warm up: Five-minute brisk walk.
Run twenty minutes.
Cool down: Walk for five minutes to bring your heart rate down, or try some of Faisal's cool-down exercises on his PMA Fitness YouTube Channel.

Block Four (Episode Date: 2 February 2020)
This block includes one run that you repeat three times during the week. This is to help train your mind to run for that amount of time, regularly.

Warm up: Five-minute brisk walk.
Run twenty minutes.
Cool down: Walk for five minutes to bring your heart rate down, or try some of Faisal's cool-down exercises on his

PMA Fitness YouTube Channel.

Block Five

Push for a harder running pace for the runs in this block; here we work on pacing with some interval training.

Run One (Episode Date: 10 February 2020)

Warm up: Five-minute brisk walk.
Run five minutes.
Walk three minutes.
Run eight minutes.
Walk three minutes.
Run five minutes.
Cool down: Walk for five minutes to bring your heart rate down, or try some of Faisal's cool-down exercises on his PMA Fitness YouTube Channel.

Run Two (Episode Date: 11 February 2020)

Warm up: Five-minute brisk walk.
Run ten minutes.
Walk three minutes.
Run ten minutes.
Cool down: Walk for five minutes to bring your heart rate down, or try some of Faisal's cool-down exercises on his PMA Fitness YouTube Channel.

Run Three (Episode Date: 13 February 2020)

Warm up: Five-minute brisk walk.
Run non-stop for twenty-five minutes.
Cool down: Walk for five minutes to bring your heart rate down, or try some of Faisal's cool-down exercises on his PMA Fitness YouTube Channel.

The Big Day (Episode Date: 14 February 2020)
Put the *RunPod* episode 'The Big Day' on and start running your first 5K – GOOD LUCK!

10K TRAINING PLAN

Now it's time to take you from 5 to 10K!
Before taking on this 10K plan, I recommend that you should be able to run a 5K comfortably in around forty minutes. This plan is an eight-week plan, but you should never feel like you can't repeat some of the weeks more than once if you like – if you feel like you need longer, that's absolutely fine!

Eight weeks to 10K
Each week, you will have the following:

✳ Three x run days

✳ One x easy 5K

* One x intervals/tempo/hill sprints

* One x long run

* Three x rest days (this can include one x recovery run after a long run day)

* One x cross-training day (yoga, stretching, swimming, strength training).

Your long run day distance will taper to Race Day:
Week One - 3K
Week Two - 5K
Week Three - 5K
Week Four - 6K
Week Five - 8K
Week Six - 9K (or 10K if you want to!)
Week Seven - 6K
Week Eight - Race Day.

Things to remember:

* You can repeat weeks if you feel you need to!

* You don't *have* to do the full 10K before Race Day – if you can run 8K, you can run 10K, but if you do want to, do so on the day of your longest planned run (not the week before your race).

* If the race route is hilly, make sure you factor in some hill sprints into your training.

* If training is interrupted by illness or holiday etc., pick up where you left off, unless the interruption is more than a week, in which case, go back a week.

For more training plans or guidance, work with a running coach, look at plans available through outlets like *Runner's World* magazine, or build your own plan in an app like Runna or Coopah.

SIXTEEN-WEEK MARATHON TRAINING PLAN

Before you start this programme, I would recommend you re-read Chapter 9 (pages 215–49) and consider whether you're ready to run a marathon right now. So many people sign up after being inspired by watching it on TV, having zero prior running experience.

If you're already running and can run 5 miles comfortably, then you should be able to build up to 26.2 miles over the course of sixteen weeks (four months). Now, that won't be true of everyone, but that can be applied most of the time. If you can't run 5 miles comfortably yet, then training may take a little longer, so perhaps allow yourself six months before Race Day instead and build up your running before you try this plan. Remember, this is a guide, not an instruction manual. You can switch days and switch the order of runs, although I would try and keep your long run to the same day or as close to it as possible. Your long run should also be the day that the race is on. So, for example, you train your body to run a long way on a Sunday, and your race will be on a Sunday. It doesn't matter if you mix it up a bit – I tend to do my long run on a Saturday or a Monday, but it gives some good structure to your training programme.

Week One – Ramping up

Tuesday – Easy run – 4 miles.

Wednesday – Five miles and in the middle run to a hill (this might even be a road near where you live), then run thirty seconds up the hill, jog down and repeat x eight.

Friday – Do a steady run at a stronger pace – 5 miles.

Sunday – Long run – 7 miles.

Week Two

Tuesday – Easy run – 4 miles.

Wednesday – Tempo run:

One mile slow

Three miles at pace (where you can't chat easily, but can breathe comfortably)

One mile slow.

Friday – Intervals:

One-mile warm up jog

Ninety seconds fast / Ninety seconds slow x eight

One-mile cool down jog.
Sunday – Long run – 9 miles.

Week Three

Tuesday – Easy run – 6 miles.
Wednesday – Five miles and in the middle run to a hill (this might even be a road near where you live), then run thirty seconds up the hill, jog down and repeat x eight.
Friday – Five miles:

One mile warm up

Three minutes fast / ninety seconds slow x five

Jog the remainder of the distance.
Sunday – Long run – 11 miles.

Week Four

Tuesday – Easy run – 7 miles.
Wednesday – Tempo run – 6 miles:

Warm up 2 miles

Pick up the pace for 3 miles

Cool down for 1 mile.
Friday – Five miles – intervals:

Warm up 2 miles

Six minutes strong run with two-minute slow run/walk x three

Cool down jog afterwards.
Sunday – Long run – 13 miles.

Week Five
Tuesday – Easy run – 8 miles.
Wednesday – Hill sprints:
   Six-mile run to a hill
   Thirty seconds uphill / jog down x ten.
Friday – Intervals:
   Warm up 2 miles easy
   Ninety seconds fast / ninety seconds slow x eight
   Cool down 1 mile.
Sunday – Long run – a fast 10K.

Week Six
Tuesday – Easy run – 9 miles.
Wednesday – Intervals:
   Warm up 2 miles
   Three minutes fast / two minutes slow x six
   Jog recovery.
Friday – Easy run – 5 miles.
Sunday – Long run – 15 miles (in the middle of the run, try to pick up the pace to marathon pace for 3 miles).

Week Seven
Tuesday – Easy run – 6 miles.
Wednesday – Fartlek – speed running (see also page 44–5):
   Warm up 2 miles
   Twelve x thirty-second sprints

In between each sprint you can jog, or walk if need be, for thirty to sixty seconds.

Friday – Intervals – 7 miles:

Warm up 2 miles

Strong run for 1 mile with two minutes rest x four

Cool down jog.

Sunday – Long run – 16 miles.

Week Eight

Tuesday – Easy run – 6 miles.

Wednesday – Fartlek – speed running:

Run thirty seconds, then slow run thirty seconds x ten.

Friday – Run at a steady pace – 4 miles.

Sunday – Long run – 18 miles.

Week Nine

Tuesday – Easy run – 8 miles.

Wednesday – Fartlek – speed running:

Six miles with sixty seconds strong runs, then slow run thirty seconds x eight in the middle.

Friday – Intervals:

Warm up 2 miles

Ninety seconds fast / ninety seconds slow x ten

Cool down 2 miles.

Sunday – Long run – 19 miles.

Week Ten

Tuesday – Easy run – 9 miles.

Wednesday – 7 miles:

Start slow and pick up pace a tiny amount every mile until 6 miles, then do a 1-mile slow jog.

Friday – Intervals:

Warm up 2 miles

Three minutes fast / two minutes slow x six

Cool down 1 mile.

Sunday – Long run – 15 miles:

Include a strong 5 miles in the middle at marathon pace.

Week Eleven

Tuesday – Steady run – 10 miles.

Wednesday – hill sprints:

Warm up 2 miles

Thirty seconds uphill / jog down x twelve

Cool down 2-mile jog.

Friday – 7-mile run:

Warm up 1 mile

Strong run 1 mile / two minutes rest x five

Cool down 1 mile.

Sunday – Long run – 20 miles – slow slow slow!

Week Twelve

Tuesday – Easy run – 9 miles.

Wednesday – Fartlek – speed running:

Six miles with thirty-second sprints / thirty seconds easy x ten.

Friday – 7-mile run:

Warm up 1 mile

Sixty seconds strong run / sixty seconds slow or walk x twenty

Jog to finish.

Sunday - Long run – 17 miles.

Do 5 miles at a stronger marathon pace in the middle.

Week Thirteen

Tuesday – Easy run – 8 miles.

Wednesday - Six miles with hill sprints – thirty seconds uphill / jog down x twelve.

Friday – Intervals:

Warm up 2 miles

Ninety seconds fast / ninety seconds slow x ten

Cool down 2 miles.

Sunday – Longest run – 21 or 22 miles, all very slow.

Week Fourteen – Tapering

Tuesday – Easy run – 6 miles.

Wednesday – 5 miles with hill sprints – thirty seconds uphill / jog down x ten.

Friday – 5 miles:

1 mile slow

3 miles marathon pace

1 mile slow.

Sunday – Long run – 15 miles.

Week Fifteen

Tuesday – Easy run – 6 miles.

Wednesday – 5 miles with hill sprints – thirty seconds uphill / jog down x ten.

Friday – 5 miles with middle 3 miles at marathon pace.

Sunday – Long run – 10 miles.

Week Sixteen – Race Week

Tuesday – Easy run – 3 miles.

Wednesday – 4 miles:

   Warm up 1 mile

   One-mile marathon pace

   Thirty seconds fast / thirty seconds slow x five

   Cool down for the remaining distance.

Friday – 2 miles – go easy easy easy!

Sunday – Race Day – TIME FOR YOUR LAP OF HONOUR!

USEFUL RESOURCES

Here's a list of some of the websites and apps I've referenced in the book that can offer you advice, support and ideas to help you on your running journey!

MOBILE APPS
Coopah – coopah.com
MapMyRun – mapmyrun.com
NHS Couch to 5k – nhs.uk/live-well/exercise/running-and-aerobic-exercises/get-running-with-couch-to-5k
Nike Run Club – nike.com/gb/nrc-app
Runkeeper – runkeeper.com
Runna – runna.com
Strava – strava.com

RUNNING TOURS
Go Running Tours – GoRunningTours.com

Running Tours – RunningTours.net
Run of a Kind Birmingham – runofakindbirmingham.com
Secret London Runs – secretlondonruns.com

COMMUNITY ACTION GROUPS
Black Girls Do Run – blackgirlsdorun.co.uk
England Athletics – englandathletics.org/find-a-club
Good Gym – goodgym.org
Good Run Guide – goodrunguide.co.uk/ClubFinder.asp
Jog Scotland – jogscotland.org.uk
Meetup running groups – meetup.com/topics/running/gb
Parkrun – parkrun.org.uk
Run Dem Crew – rundemcrew.com
Run Talk Run – runtalkrun.com
Run Together – runtogether.co.uk
This Girl Runs – thisgirlruns.club/find-a-club

ONLINE COMMUNITIES
Lonely Goat – lonelygoat.com
Slow AF Run Club – slowafrunclub.com
This Mum Runs – thismumruns.co.uk

VIRTUAL RACES
TCS London Marathon MyWay – tcslondonmarathon.com
/the-event/virtual-marathon
Virtual Runner UK – virtualrunneruk.com

ALTERNATIVE RACES

Dragon's Back Race – dragonsbackrace.com

Inflatable 5k – ukrunningevents.co.uk/events/inflatable-5k

Marathon des Sables – marathondessables.co.uk

Marathon du Médoc – marathondumedoc.com/en

Polar Circle Marathon – polar-circle-marathon.com

Race for Life – raceforlife.cancerresearchuk.org/find-an-event

Race the Train – racethetrain.com

Run Alton Towers – runaltontowers.com

Spartan – spartan.com

Spartathlon – spartathlon.gr/en

Tough Mudder – toughmudder.co.uk

Walt Disney World Marathon Weekend – rundisney.com

Whole Earth Man v Horse – green-events.co.uk/?mvh_main

Endnotes

1   https://www.sportengland.org/news/childrens-activity-levels-recover-pre-pandemic-levels

2   https://www.theguardian.com/society/2023/jul/18/people-who-cram-weeks-exercise-into-two-days-reap-similar-heart-benefits-study

3   https://www.womensrunning.co.uk/news/national-womens-running-survey-2022-harassment-run

4   https://what3words.com/products/what3words-app

5   https://www.vernonwilliamsmd.com/News-Updates/2022/June/This-Is-Exactly-What-Happens-to-Your-Brain-Durin.aspx#:~:text=2%20to%204%20hours%3A%20A,4%20hours%20after%20your%20workout
    https://www.healthline.com/health/runners-high
    https://marathonhandbook.com/runners-high/

6   https://www.pnas.org/doi/10.1073/pnas.1514996112

7   https://www.ncbi.nlm.nih.gov/pmc/articles/PMC7663387/

8   https://www.ncbi.nlm.nih.gov/pmc/articles/PMC2817271/

9   https://www.ncbi.nlm.nih.gov/pmc/articles/PMC7663387/

10 https://www.theguardian.com/lifeandstyle/2023/jul/24/slow-running-revolution-sexy-pace-enjoy-the-race

11 https://www.telegraph.co.uk/health-fitness/wellbeing/sleep/how-to-sleep-like-a-tennis-champion/

12 https://www.realhomes.com/news/venus-williams-ghost-bed-sleep-tips

13 https://www.runnersworld.com/uk/news/a28299379/kipchoge-sleeps-for-this-many-hours-every-day/

14 https://yougov.co.uk/topics/health/articles-reports/2022/06/29/yougov-sleep-study-part-one-sleeping-patterns

15   https://pubmed.ncbi.nlm.nih.gov/20861519/

16 https://www.runandbecome.com/running-training-advice/low-heart-rate-training

17 https://www.runnersworld.com/uk/health/injury/a41351417/cramp-in-calf/